Leiomyoma

Edited by Hassan Abduljabbar

Published in London, United Kingdom

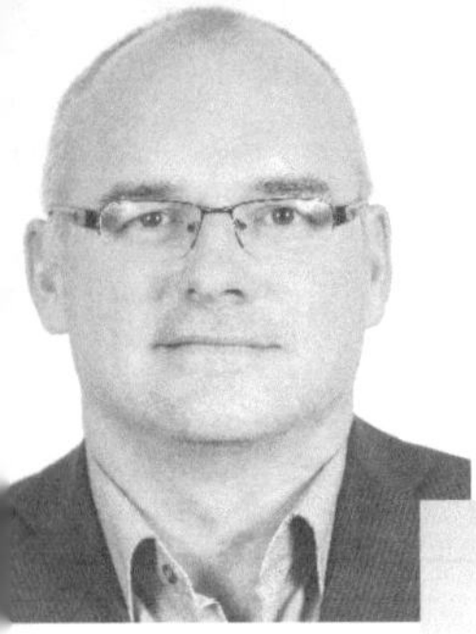
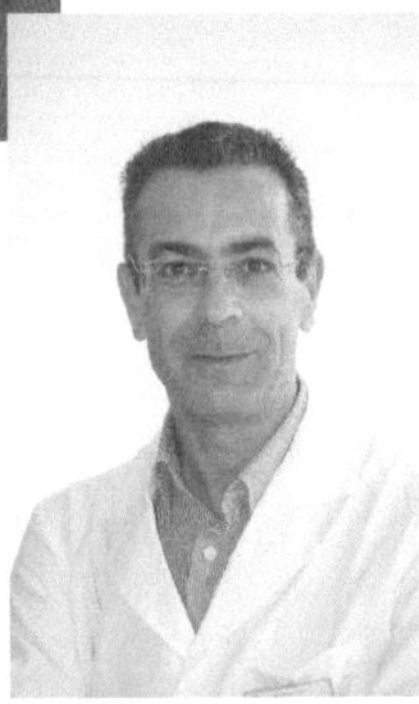
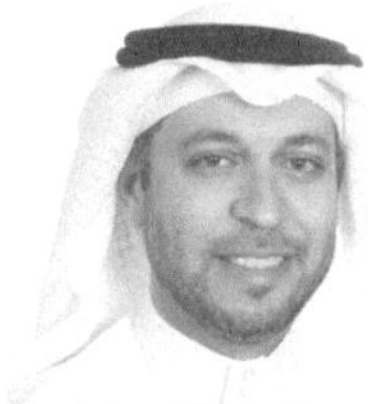
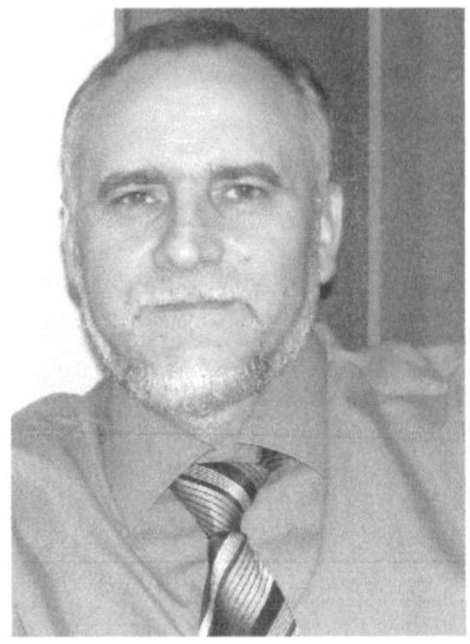
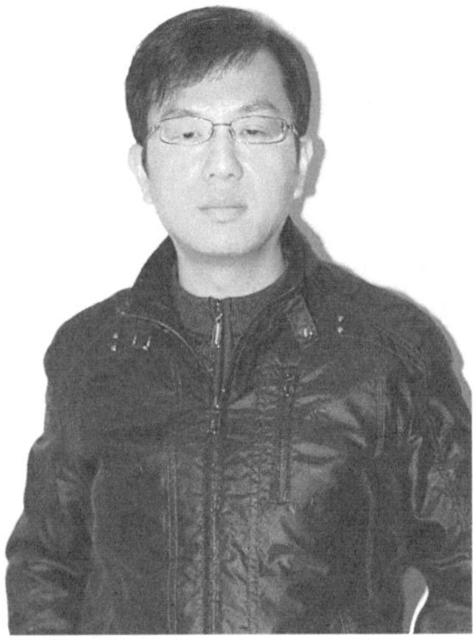
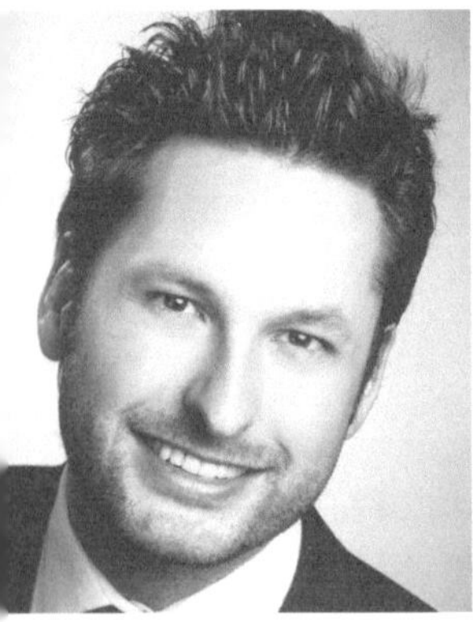
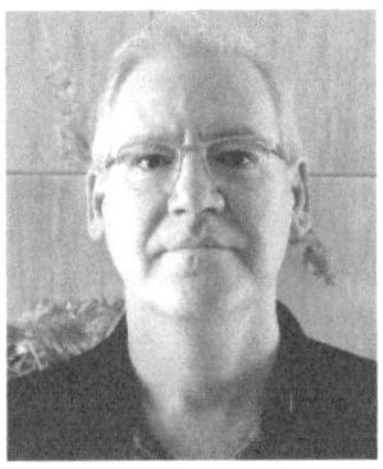

IntechOpen

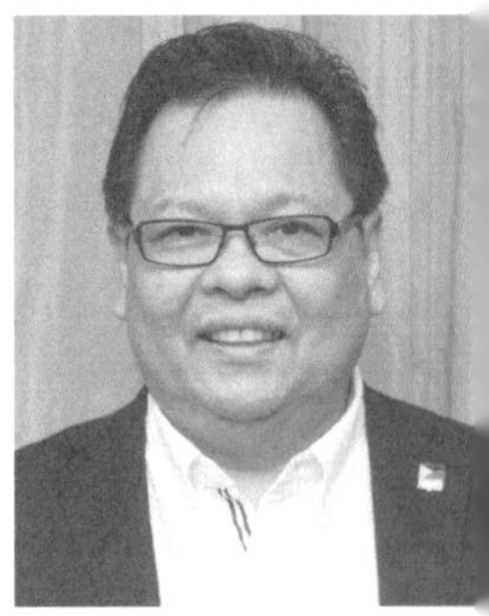
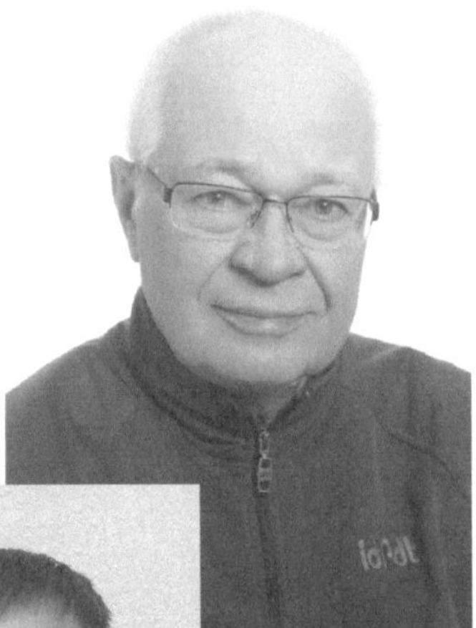
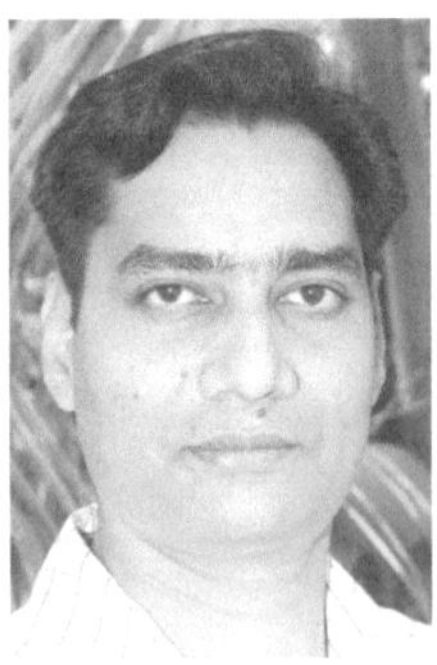
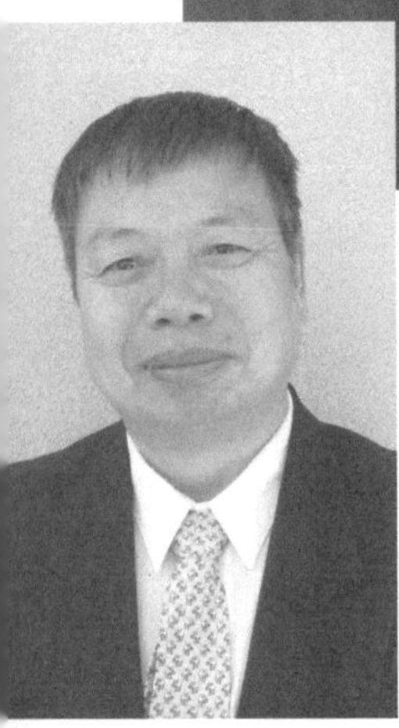
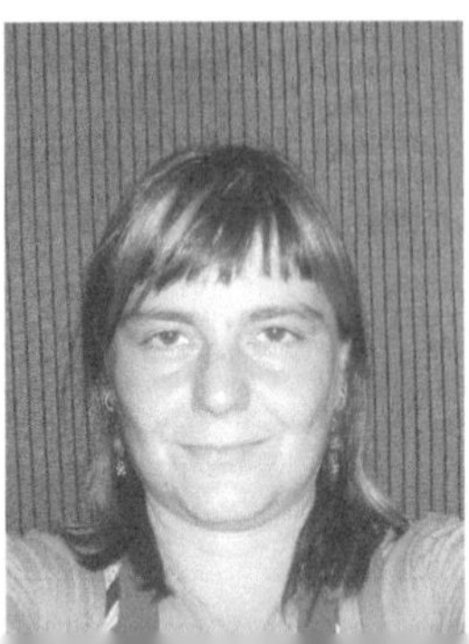
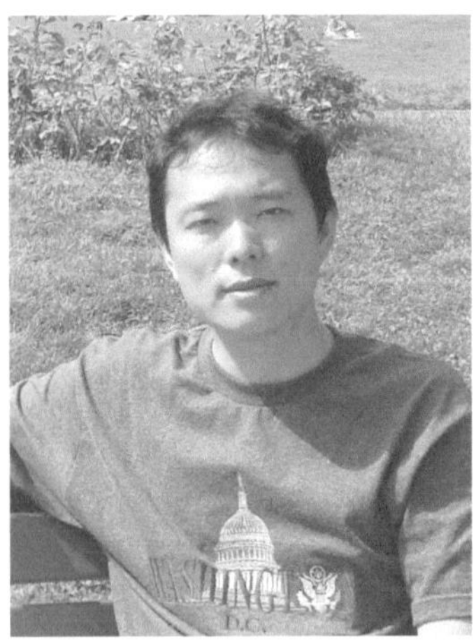

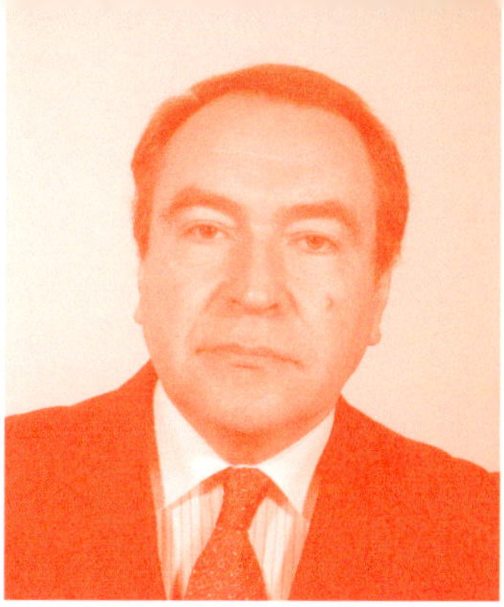

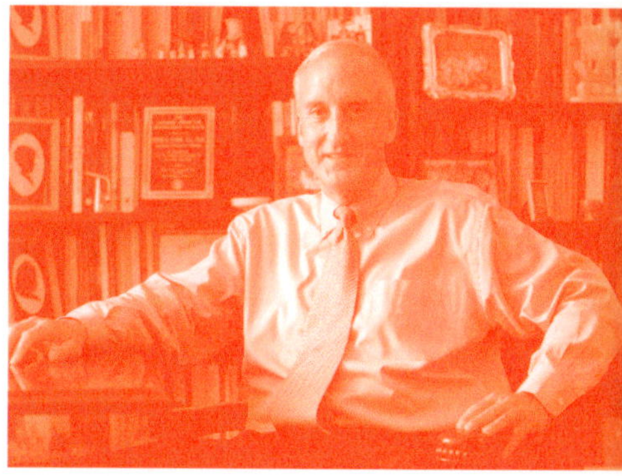

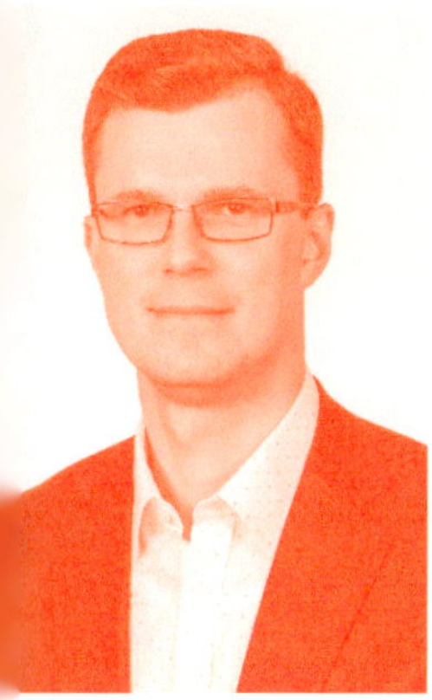

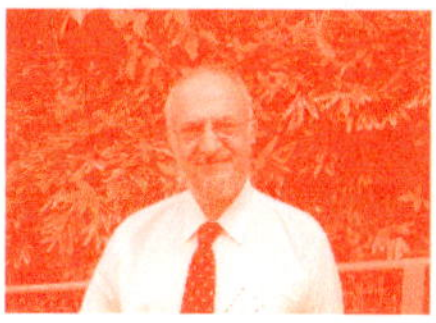

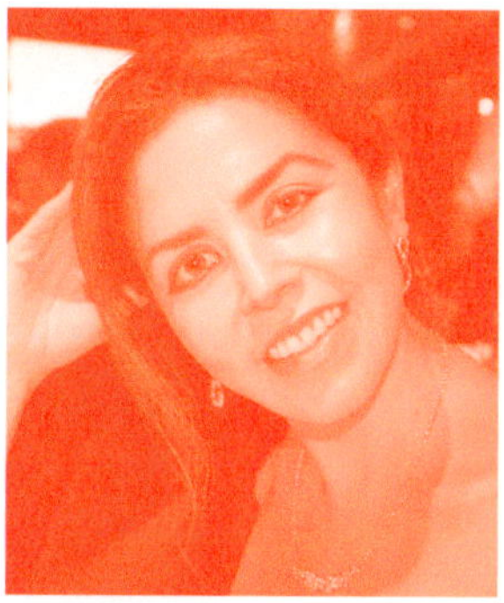

Supporting open minds since 2005

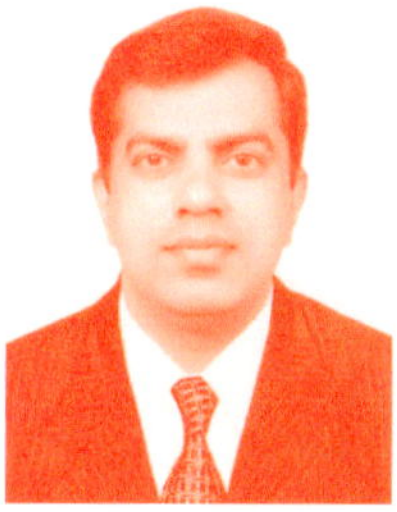

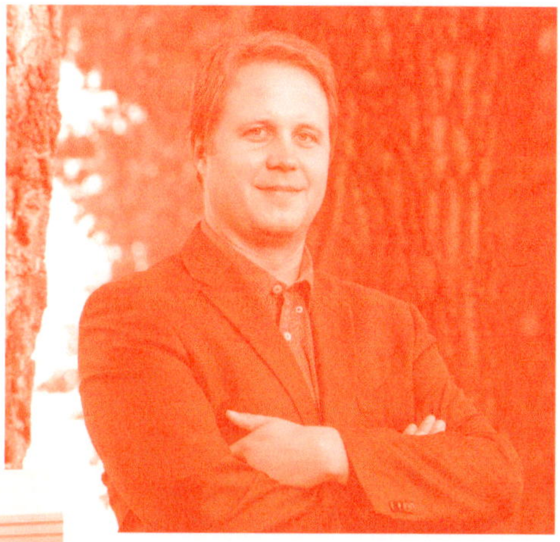

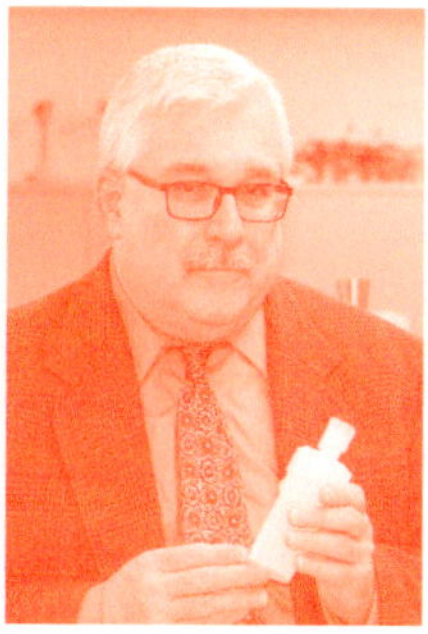

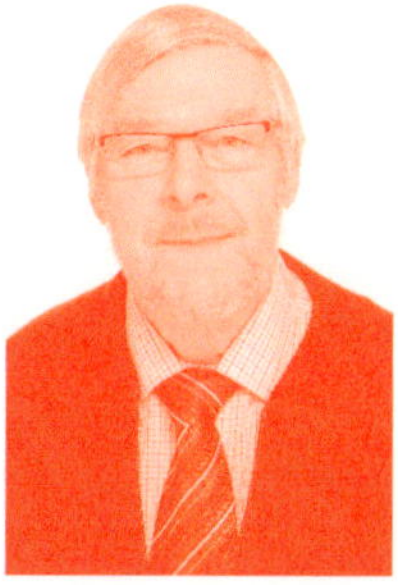

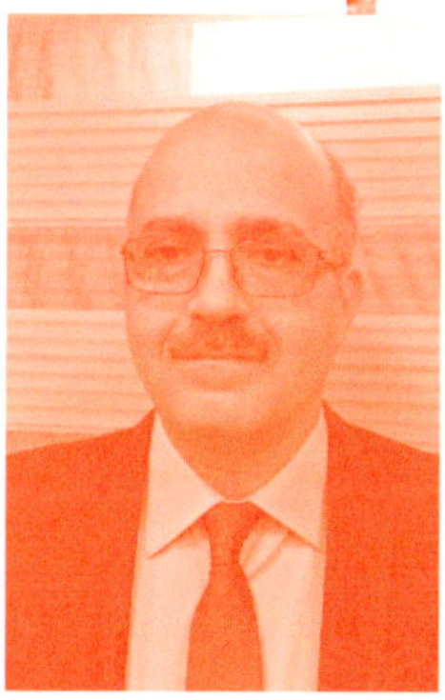

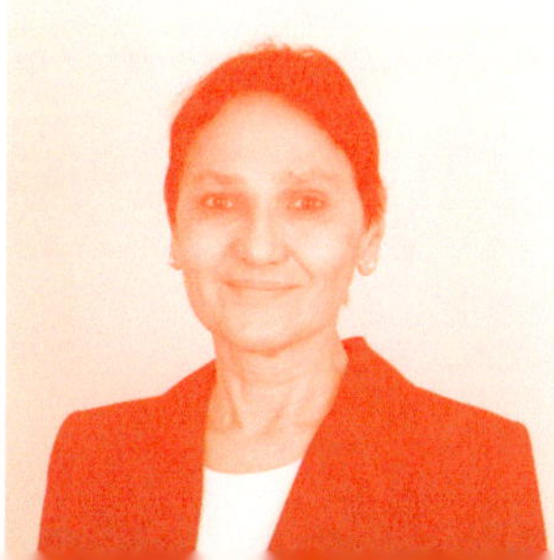

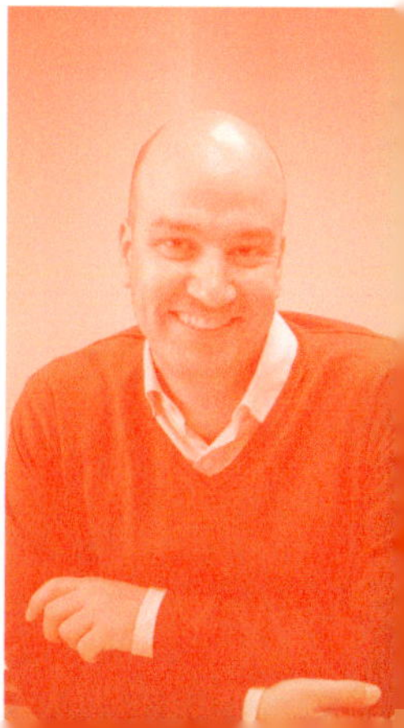

Leiomyoma
http://dx.doi.org/10.5772/intechopen.77799
Edited by Hassan Abduljabbar

Contributors
Felix Oindi, Mukaindo Mwaniki, Hassan S Abduljabbar, Razvan Socolov, Ioana Pavaleanu, Demetra Socolov, Mona Akad, Ciprian Ilea, Chrisostomos Sofoudis, Arash Fereydooni, Naiem Nassiri, Said Izreig

First published in London, United Kingdom, 2020 by IntechOpen
IntechOpen is the global imprint of INTECHOPEN LIMITED, registered in England and Wales, registration number: 11086078, 7th floor, 10 Lower Thames Street, London, EC3R 6AF, United Kingdom
Printed in Croatia

British Library Cataloguing-in-Publication Data
A catalogue record for this book is available from the British Library

Additional hard and PDF copies can be obtained from orders@intechopen.com

Leiomyoma
Edited by Hassan Abduljabbar
p. cm.
Print ISBN 978-1-78985-423-7
Online ISBN 978-1-78985-424-4
eBook (PDF) ISBN 978-1-78985-830-3

Meet the editor

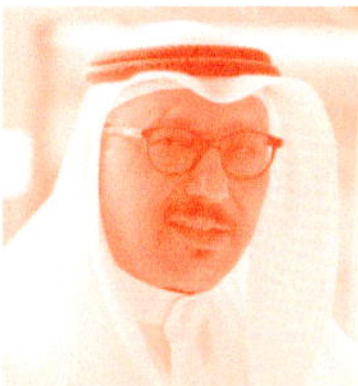

Professor Hassan S. Abduljabbar, MD, FRCSC, American Board Diplomat, is a professor of the Medical College, King Abdulaziz University, and President of the Saudi Society of Obstetrics and Gynecology. He graduated from King Abdulaziz University, College of Medicine and Allied Health Sciences, Jeddah, Saudi Arabia, in June 1980, with an MD degree (overall grade: excellent secondary honor). He obtained his FRCS(C) degree at the Royal College of Physicians and Surgeons of Canada in November 1986 after 4 years of training at the University of Western Ontario. Then, in December 1988, he obtained American Board of Obstetrics and Gynecology certification. He was Chairman of the Department of Obstetrics and Gynecology, and is now President of the Saudi Society of Obstetrics and Gynecology. He is a referee of many international scientific medical journals. He is an examiner of master's degrees and PhD degrees as well as a member of the Saudi and Arabia board of examination. He writes weekly scientific subjects in local newspapers (Al Bilad). His publications in local and international journals exceed 50 articles, and he is the editor of two books—Steroid Basics (Open Access Books—IntechOpen) and Steroid Clinical (Open Access Books—IntechOpen)—and the author of a 100 Multiple-Choice Questions book for medical students. He has published four books in the Arabic, Aafaq 1 and 2, stem cell and breast cancer medical subject for nonmedical personal (in Arabic, 2006).

Contents

Preface

This book introduces an important subject, and aims to explore one of the most common pathologic abnormalities of the female genital tract: leiomyoma of the uterus, which is a benign tumor of the smooth muscle.

The occurrence of uterine leiomyoma increases with age, is found in 20–50% of women older than 30 years, but is rare in children and post-menopausal women.

Uterine leiomyoma results in masses associated with a variety of gynecologic problems, the most prominent of which are asymptomatic pelvic mass and abnormal vaginal bleeding.

The majority of women are asymptomatic, but may suffer pain and heavy vaginal bleeding, or have other urinary symptoms. Uterine fibroids can also cause sexual dysfunction and dyspareunia, infertility, and recurrent pregnancy loss.

The etiology of uterine fibroids is unclear, but may be a hormone-related or estrogen-dependent disease. Risk factors include race, age, genetics, and high BMI (obesity), and may be related to diet especially eating meat.

Diagnosis by clinical history and physical examination, pelvic examination, ultrasound pelvis and CT scan, and MRI are helpful.

Major complications can occur if the uterine fibroids are caused by iron deficiency due to heavy monthly blood loss, which can cause fatigue, and sometimes transfusion is needed due to severe anemia.

Fibroids may or may not interfere with fertility and pregnancy. However, submucosal fibroids could cause infertility or recurrent pregnancy loss.

Fibroids may also raise the risk of pregnancy complications, such as fetal growth restriction, preterm delivery, and placental abruption. Red degeneration of fibroids during pregnancy can cause severe abdominal pain.

Can fibroids be prevented? Researchers have admitted that little scientific evidence is available on how to prevent fibroids. Uterine fibroids may be prevented, and only a small percentage of these tumors require treatment.

Healthy lifestyle choices, such as maintaining a normal weight and eating fruits and vegetables, may be able to decrease the risk of having fibroids.

Research suggests that using hormonal contraceptives may be associated with a lower risk of fibroids.

Management can be medical hormonal or non-hormonal, open surgical, endoscopic, or uterine artery embolization.

Hassan Abduljabbar
King Abdul Aziz University,
Saudi Arabia

Section 1

Clinical Presentation

Chapter 1

Uterine Fibroids: Clinical Presentation

Felix J.M. Oindi and Mukaindo A. Mwaniki

Abstract

The signs and symptoms of leiomyoma are varied. Most patients with uterine fibroids are asymptomatic and require no treatment. This is especially so in patients with small subserosal and intramural leiomyomas. Such patients may have the leiomyomas discovered incidentally during workup for other medical condition such as pregnancy. Some of them are also incidentally discovered in hysterectomy specimens for other pelvic masses. The common symptoms associated with leiomyomas include menorrhagia, pelvic pain or pressure, and subfertility. These symptoms vary from one patient to another and do not necessarily correlate to the size of the fibroids. Abdomino-pelvic examination may be normal if the fibroids are small. However, findings of a suprapubic mass and tenderness are not an uncommon finding for bigger myomas.

Keywords: leiomyoma, asymptomatic, menorrhagia, pelvic pain, pressure symptoms

1. Clinical presentation of uterine fibroids

Uterine fibroids present with a variety of signs and symptoms. The majority of women are asymptomatic, and the fibroid masses often remain undiagnosed [1]. Among such women, the myomas may be discovered during investigation for other conditions [2–4]. More than 50% of patients with uterine fibroids have no symptoms. This is common for small myomas especially when subserosal. For instance, a patient would be discovered to have fibroids during an antenatal ultrasound assessment of the foetus or during imaging for assessment of other pelvic pathologies such as appendicitis or ovarian masses. Fibroids would also be discovered in hysterectomy specimens done for other gynaecological conditions such as cervical and ovarian malignancies.

Among symptomatic women, abnormal uterine bleeding is the commonest complaint [1]. This could be described as heavy, prolonged, bleeding between menses or painful bleeding. The other symptoms associated with leiomyomas include pelvic pain, pelvic pressure and subfertility.

2. Abnormal uterine bleeding

Menorrhagia, defined as an increase in the amount of blood loss per month, is the most common symptom of uterine fibroids [1]. Majority of women with fibroids describe an increase in the amount of menstrual flow with some either needing to use more pads than before, using 'heavier pads' or even using both a tampon and a pad simultaneously. Some report flooding whereby the bleeding flows beyond the containing pad/tampon. This kind of bleeding may cause anaemia, one of the commonest complications of menorrhagia.

The mechanism by which fibroids cause menorrhagia has not been clearly established. However, a few theories have been fronted [4]. These include an increase in the endometrial surface area especially from fibroids with a submucosal component. Heavy menstrual flow may also result from increased vascularity of the uterus due the increased endothelial growth factors, principally VEGF [3, 5]. Other probable mechanisms include interference with normal uterine contractility and endometrial ulceration over the myomas [6]. Menorrhagia may also result from venous congestion due to compression of venous plexus within the myometrium and endometrium with resultant endometrial venule ectasia leading to profuse bleeding.

Menorrhagia since menarche implies a possibility of other mechanisms of menorrhagia [7]. These patients should be evaluated for coagulopathies as up to 13% may have von Willebrand disease. Occurrence of myomas in such patients serves to worsen the already existing heavy uterine bleeding. These patients should be evaluated and managed by a multidisciplinary team including physicians, haematologists and gynaecologists.

Other bleeding abnormalities commonly reported include prolonged bleeding, bleeding between menses, frequent periods and irregular and unpredictable periods [1]. Intermenstrual bleeding is more likely for cervical fibroids especially when close to the endo-cervical canal. Ulceration of fibroids with a submucosal component may also cause intermenstrual bleeding.

3. Pelvic pain

This is a less common symptom than abnormal uterine bleeding, and patients rarely present with pain as the sole complaint [4, 6]. Intramural fibroids may present with dysmenorrhea alongside the menorrhagia. However, the dysmenorrhea may not always be associated with menorrhagia. Degenerative changes, common in pregnancy, may also cause pelvic pain. This is usually managed conservatively by analgesics and rest. Dyspareunia is less common.

Some patients may present with chronic pelvic pain and dyspareunia [1].

Acute pain may result from torsion of a pedunculated myoma's pedicle, incarceration of a myoma within the pelvis or even cervical dilatation by a submucous myoma [4]. Cervical torsion may result in catastrophic intra-abdominal bleeding necessitating emergency laparotomy/laparoscopy.

4. Pressure-/bulk-related symptoms

Depending on the size and location, uterine fibroids may compress the urinary bladder or rectum [4, 6]. Compression of the urinary bladder may present with urinary frequency, difficulty emptying the bladder and even acute urinary retention. When large, myomas may cause ureteric obstruction and hydronephrosis, which is more common on the right.

Fibroids can also place pressure on the rectum and cause constipation.

Patients may also present with feeling of an abdominal mass without any apparent menstrual disturbances or pain. Such patients may be suspected during examination for other conditions. Large fibroids may also cause compression of the inferior vena cava leading to possible deep venous thrombosis of the lower extremities.

DOI: http://dx.doi.org/10.5772/intechopen.88473

5. Reproductive challenges

Patients with fibroids may present with subfertility [6, 8]. As the occurrence of both uterine fibroids and subfertility increases with age, so does the risk of aneuploidy and pregnancy loss. Therefore, the actual impact of fibroids on fertility is difficult to ascertain. Submucosal and intramural fibroids distorting the uterine cavity compromise fertility. Depending on the number, size and location, fibroids may distort the overall uterine anatomy and compromise fertility. Removal of such fibroids may enhance fertility. Up to 60% of patients have been shown to conceive spontaneously upon myomectomy.

Fibroids may also increase the rates of first and second trimester miscarriages [9]. They have also been implicated as a cause of recurrent pregnancy loss.

6. Pregnancy-related complications

Fibroids may present with acute pain in pregnancy due to degenerative changes [6, 8]. They may also cause premature rupture of membranes, preterm labour, abruption placenta, malpresentations, foetal growth restriction and increased operative deliveries. Leiomyomas may also cause postpartum haemorrhage, retained placenta and even puerperal sepsis.

Author details

Felix J.M. Oindi* and Mukaindo A. Mwaniki
Department of Obstetrics and Gynaecology, Aga Khan University Hospital, Nairobi, Kenya

*Address all correspondence to: droindi@gmail.com

References

[1] Zimmermann A, Bernuit D, Gerlinger C, Schaefers M, Geppert K. Prevalence, symptoms and management of uterine fibroids: An international internet-based survey of 21,746 women. BMC Women's Health. 2012;**12**:6

[2] Divakar H. Asymptomatic uterine fibroids. Best Practice & Research. Clinical Obstetrics & Gynaecology. 2008;**22**(4):643-654

[3] Bulun SE. Uterine fibroids. The New England Journal of Medicine. 2013;**369**(14):1344-1355

[4] Gupta S, Jose J, Manyonda I. Clinical presentation of fibroids. Best Practice & Research. Clinical Obstetrics & Gynaecology. 2008;**22**(4):615-626

[5] Flake GP, Andersen J, Dixon D. Etiology and pathogenesis of uterine leiomyomas: A review. Environmental Health Perspectives. 2003;**111**(8):1037-1054

[6] Parker WH. Etiology, symptomatology, and diagnosis of uterine myomas. Fertility and Sterility. 2007;**87**(4):725-736

[7] Munro MG, Lukes AS. Abnormal uterine bleeding and underlying hemostatic disorders: Report of a consensus process. Fertility and Sterility. 2005;**84**(5):1335-1337

[8] Farquhar C. Do uterine fibroids cause infertility and should they be removed to increase fertility? BMJ (Clinical Research Edition). 2009;**b126**:338

[9] Al-Hendy A, Myers ER, Stewart E. Uterine fibroids: Burden and unmet medical need. Seminars in Reproductive Medicine. 2017;**35**(6):473-480

Chapter 2

Bizarre Leiomyoma of the Uterus: Therapeutic Mapping

Chrisostomos Sofoudis

Abstract

Leiomyomas represent the most common type of benign tumors of the female genital tract. Assiduous preoperative imaging findings reflect proper therapeutic mapping. In cases of female patients of reproductive age, the ultimate goal remains the fertility preservation and the quality of life of the patient. According to recent bibliography, bizarre leiomyomas remain a controversial issue regarding the preoperative and postoperative therapeutic mapping. Giant cells with pleomorphic nuclei and little or no mitotic activity compose the microscopic analysis of such lesions. Multidisciplinary approach is mandatory in order to establish ultimate diagnosis and treatment. Bizarre leiomyomas still represent a gray scale among the whole scientific community.

Keywords: bizarre myomas, uterus, fertility preservation

1. Introduction

The incidence of uterine fibroid tumors increases as women grow older, and they may occur in more than 30% of women 40–60 years of age (**Figure 1**). Risk factors include null parity, obesity, family history, black race, and hypertension.

Many tumors are asymptomatic and may be diagnosed incidentally. Many studies have indicated the proper therapeutic mapping in cases of nulliparous young patients.

Therapeutic strategy is strongly accompanied with age and fertility capacity of the patient. In cases of degenerated uterine fibroids in nulliparous patients, laparoscopic approach represents the gold standard of surgical confrontation.

In reproductive age women, 15–30% of these tumors are responsible for menstrual disorders, anemia due to perfuse uterine bleeding, pelvic pain, pregnancy loss, rarely preterm birth, and percentage of infertility [1].

In order to establish a proper diagnosis and treatment, especially in women of reproductive age, there is a classification of uterine fibroids [2].

Major categories consist of submucosal, intramural, subserosal, and others (cervical, parasitic) (**Table 1**).

Many factors affect the therapeutic mapping of uterine myomas. Age of the patient, gynecologic or obstetrical history, previous surgical procedures and fertility preservation.

Uterine fibroids consist of smooth muscular tissue with always the possibility of malignant transformation. Tumor size and anatomic location are strongly accompanied with assiduous therapeutic strategy.

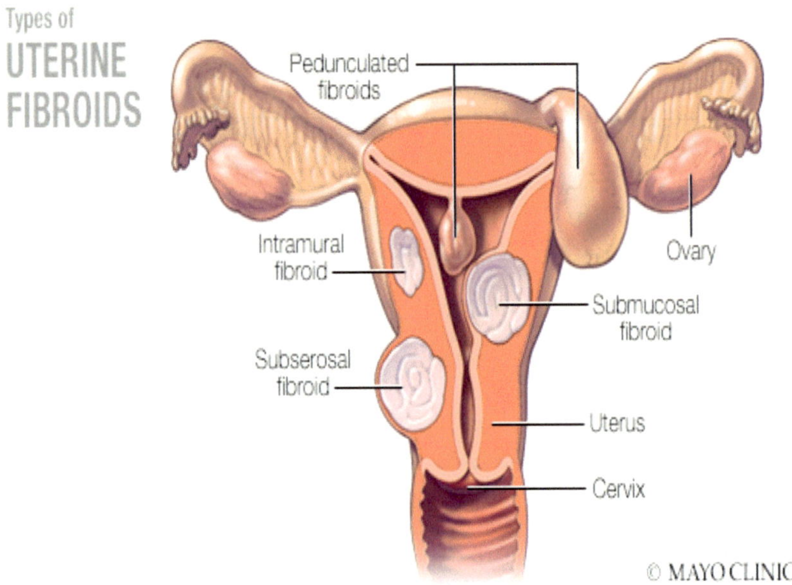

Figure 1.
Uterine fibroids. newsnetwork.mayoklinic.org.

Polyp		Coagulopathy
Adenomyosis	Submucosal	Ovulatory dysfunction
Leiomyoma →	Other	Endometrial
Malignancy and hyperplasia		Iatrogenic
		Not yet classified

Leiomyoma subclassification system

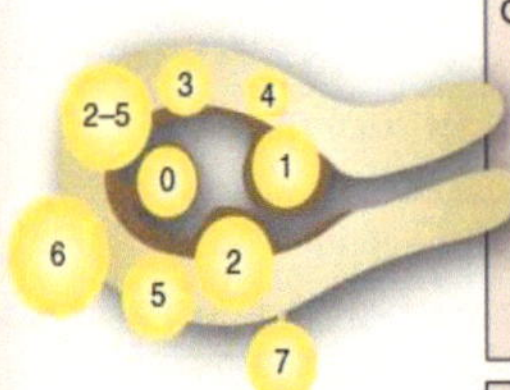

Submucosal	0	Pedunculated intracavitary
	1	<50% intramural
	2	≥50% intramural
Other	3	Contacts endometrium; 100% intramural
	4	Intramural
	5	Subserosal ≥50% intramural
	6	Subserosal <50% intramural
	7	Subserosal pedunculated
	8	Other (specify e.g., cervical, parasitic)
Hybrid leiomyomas (impact both endometrium and serosa)	Two numbers are listed separated by a hyphen. By convention, the first refers to the relationship with the endometrium, while the second refers to the relationship to the serosa. One example below:	
	2–5	Submucosal and subserosal, each with less than half the diameters in the endometrial and peritoneal cavities, respectively

Medscape   Source: Women's Health © 2014 Future Medicine Ltd

Table 1.
Classification of uterine fibroids. Women's Health 2014. Future Medicine Ltd.

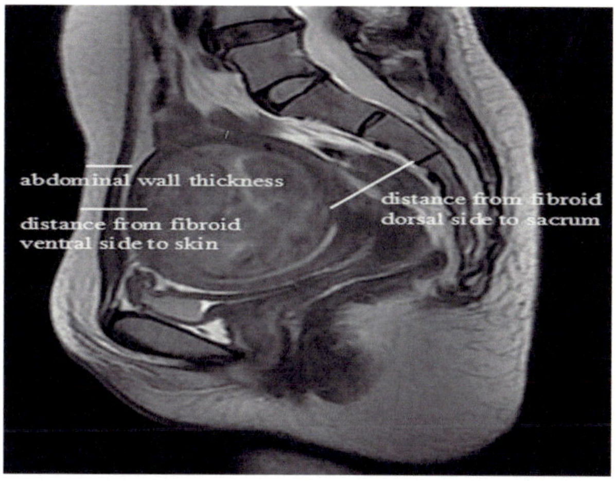

Figure 2.
Abdominal MRI with enlarged uterine fibroid depiction. Researchgate.net.

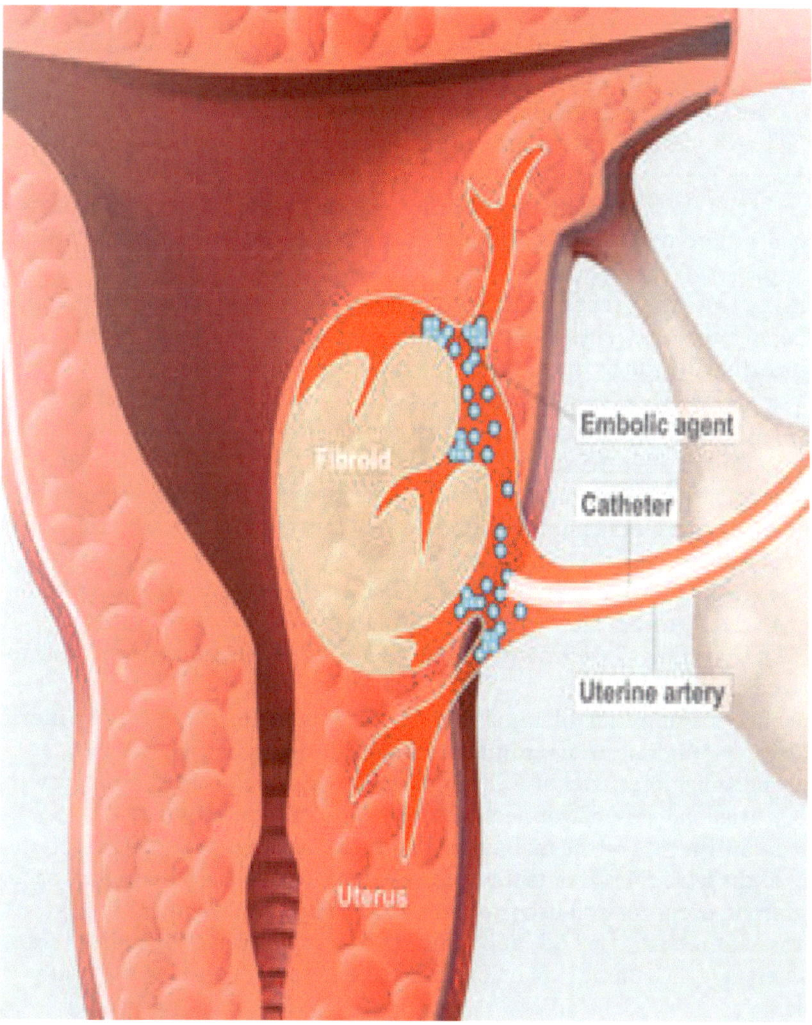

Figure 3.
Uterine fibroid embolization. Interventionalnews.com.

Transvaginal ultrasonography reflects the first preoperative procedure, depending on the physician's experience and technical sufficiency of the ultrasound machine.

Imaging findings as areas of cystic degeneration, enlarged and asymmetric vascularization, papillary protrusions, and possibly increased tumor markers as Ca-125/Ca 15-3/Ca 19-9 reveal preoperative procedures of malignant metaplasia [3].

In such cases, abdominal MRI can, without a doubt, guide the preoperative management [4] (**Figure 2**).

In order to avoid diffuse menorrhagia and procedures of diffuse intravascular coagulation, an appropriate solution consists of uterine fibroid embolization [5]. With the use of colloid substances, we can lead to fibroid necrosis and cell apoptosis (**Figure 3**).

There are cases after fibroid surgical dissection and abdominal or vaginal hysterectomy where the histopathologic evaluation confirms bizarre myomas. The dilemma is controversial especially in cases of female patients of reproductive age. The ultimate goal remains fertility preservation of such patients.

2. Discussion

All mentioned scientific guidelines reflect the pathway from general depictions of uterine anatomy and physiology to specific fibroid pathology.

Many authors complete their monograph concerning uterine fibroids. They described several tumors with similar macroscopic view as uterine fibroid, but microscopically they include large multinucleated tumor cells.

After WHO (World Health Organization) classification bizarre leiomyomas presented as fibroids with giant cells with pleomorphic nuclei and little or no mitotic activity [6].

In many cases they represent a histologic gray zone concerning the therapeutic mapping in female patients of reproductive age.

Before final diagnosis is established, assiduous examination of the specimen is mandatory focusing on terms of atypia or necrosis (simple, moderate, or severe).

Along with genetic predisposition and ovarian hormone stimulation, many growth factors are identified.

Besides genetic predisposition and ovarian hormones that play a major role in tumor expansion, a large number of growth factors have also been identified which favor expansion.

These are insulin-like growth factor (IGF), epidermal growth factor (EGF) and platelet-derived growth factor (PDGF), transforming growth factor beta (TGF beta), and basic fibroblast growth factor (BFGF) [7]. These may have a role to play in tumor expansion.

The major differential dilemma remains the establishment of bizarre uterine myomas versus endometrial stromal sarcoma (ESS) (**Figure 4**).

The main characteristics of ESS consist of infiltrative myometrium growth and vascular invasion, presence of necrotic areas, and mitotic activity [8].

Due to infiltration of the myometrial basal membrane, surgical dissection after staging of the lesion represents the gold standard. Multidisciplinary approach is mandatory in order to establish proper postoperative treatment.

In cases of metastatic ESS, neoadjuvant therapy or series of radiotherapy will understage the tumor expansion and make the tumor staging surgically feasible.

On the other hand, patients with positive progesterone or estrogen receptors (ER+, PR+), can be treated postoperatively with hormonal agents such as progestogens [9].

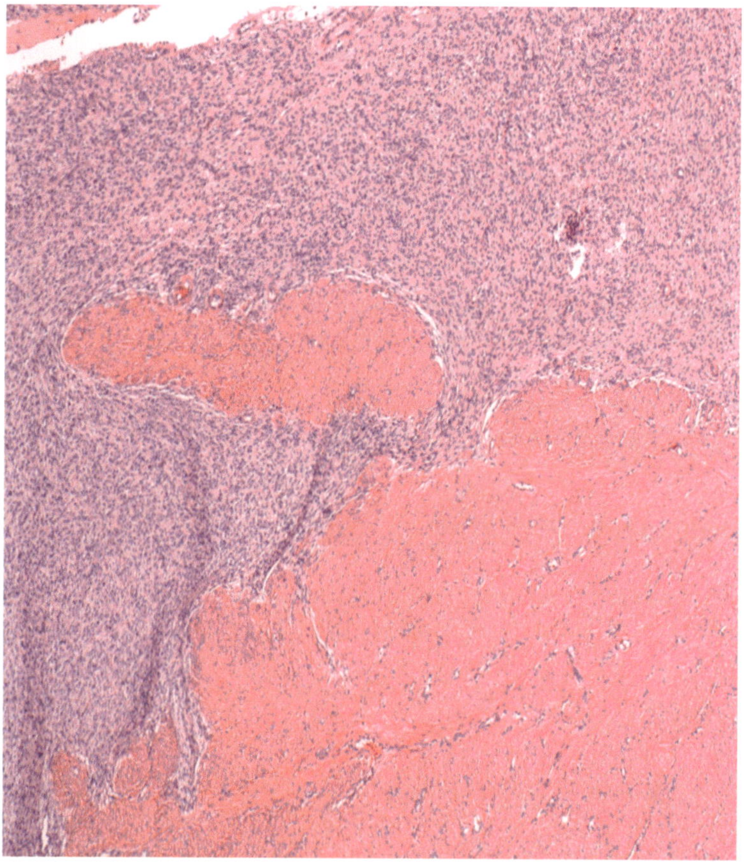

Figure 4.
Endometrial stromal sarcoma. H&E stain. Wikipedia.

Ki-67 as exceptional biomarker is strongly accompanied with proliferative activity and presence of necrotic areas. Many conducted studies have adjusted Ki-6 and successful postoperative management.

In primary stages of the lesion, fertility preservation in female patients of reproductive age remains a controversial dilemma [10].

The impact of bizarre leiomyoma on fertility is not well known. Bizarre leiomyoma consists of a rare entity composing pleomorphic or symplastic cells which require assiduous histopathologic evaluation.

If fertility preservation is not required, the standard surgical intervention for bizarre leiomyoma that shows a benign clinical course is a simple hysterectomy [11, 12].

Due to rare incidence of bizarre myomas, in cases of female patients of reproductive age with ultimate scope the fertility preservation, simple myomectomy as the gold standard remains a controversial issue.

Etiology concerning this issue depends on the identification difficulty during myomectomy between specimen surgical borders and myometrium. After histopathologic evaluation and not clear surgical margins, there is an increased incidence of tumor recurrence [13].

On the other hand, surgical treatment with dissection part of the associated myometrium, can lead in a future pregnancy, to spontaneously membrane rupture and episodes of preterm birth.

Precise scientific evaluation of current bibliography, focusing on optimal treatment in patients of reproductive age, reveals a lack of scientific guidelines.

The ultimate scope of the above presentation reflects the stimulus of completion and composition new conducted studies, which will guide assiduously and clear all controversial issues.

Bizarre uterine myomas, as rare entity, still represent a gray area among the whole scientific society.

3. Conclusion

Bizarre uterine fibroids represent a controversial scientific zone in the current bibliography. More studies must be conducted in order to establish proper diagnosis and treatment.

Multidisciplinary approach is mandatory in cases of patients of reproductive age. The ultimate goal remains in such cases, always fertility preservation.

Acknowledgements

Significant role to the completion of this book chapter, exploration and searching throughout medical data bases such as PubMed and Cochrane database.

Disclosure of interest

The author declares no financial procedure with respect to this manuscript.

Author details

Chrisostomos Sofoudis
Department of Obstetrics and Gynecology, Konstandopoulio General Hospital, Athens, Greece

*Address all correspondence to: chrisostomos.sofoudis@gmail.com

References

[1] Bulun S. Uterine fibroids. New England Journal of Medicine. 2013;**369**:1344-1355

[2] Laughlin-Tommaso SK, Hesley GK, Hopkins MR, Brandt KR, Zhu Y, Stewart EA. Clinical limitations of the International Federation of Gynecology and Obstetrics (FIGO) classification of uterine fibroids. International Journal of Gynaecology and Obstetrics. 2017;**139**(2):143-148

[3] Chander B, Shekhar S. Osseous metaplasia in leiomyoma: A first in a uterine leiomyoma. Journal of Cancer Research and Therapeutics. 2015;**11**(3):661

[4] Nakai G, Yamada T, Hamada T, et al. Pathological findings of uterine tumors preoperatively diagnosed as red degeneration of leiomyoma by MRI. Abdominal Radiology (New York). 2017;**42**(7):1825-1831

[5] Duvnjak S, Ravn P, Green A, Andersen PE. Uterine fibroid embolization with acrylamido polyvinyl microspheres: Prospective 12-month clinical and MRI follow-up study. Acta Radiologica. 2017;**58**(8):952-958

[6] Downes KA, William RH. Bizarre leiomyomas of the uterus. A comprehensive pathologic study of 24 cases with long term follow up. The American Journal of Surgical Pathology. 1997;**21**:1261-1270

[7] Srinivasan R, Saraiya U. Recurrent fibroids. Journal of Obstetrics and Gynecology of India. 2004;**54**: 363-366

[8] Chang KL, Grabtree GS, Lim-Tan Kempson RL, Hendrickson MR. Primary uterine endometrial stromal neoplasms. A clinicopathologic study of 117 cases. The American Journal of Surgical Pathology. 1994;**18**:635-658

[9] Yang KH, Shin JA, Jung JH, et al. A case of metastatic low-grade endometrial stromal sarcoma treated with letrozole after ovarian ablation by radiotherapy. Cancer Research and Treatment. 2015;**47**(4):958-962

[10] Xie W, Cao D, Yang J, Jiang X, et al. Fertility-sparing surgery for patients with low-grade endometrial stromal sarcoma. Oncotarget. 2017;**8**(6):10602-10608

[11] Solomon LA, Schimp VL, Ali-Fehmi R, Diamond MP, Munkarah AR. Clinical update of smooth muscle tumors of the uterus. Journal of Minimally Invasive Gynecology. 2005;**12**:401-408

[12] Sung CO, Ahn G, Song SY, et al. Atypical leiomyomas of the uterus with long-term follow-up after myomectomy with immunohistochemical analysis for p16INK4A, p53, Ki-67, estrogen receptors, and progesterone receptors. International Journal of Gynecological Pathology. 2009;**28**:529-534

[13] Toledo G, Oliva E. Smooth muscle tumors of the uterus: A practical approach. Archives of Pathology & Laboratory Medicine. 2008;**132**:595-605

Section 2

Management

Chapter 3

Different Surgical Techniques for Management of Leiomyoma

Hassan S.O. Abduljabbar and Abdullah K. Agabawi

Abstract

The objective is to review the methods of treatment for all cases diagnosed as leiomyoma at Tertiary Teaching Hospital. This is a retrospective study on the medical files of all cases diagnosed as leiomyoma at King Abdulaziz University Hospital. It is a teaching hospital with a capacity of 800 beds in total and 180 beds in the Department of Obstetrics and Gynecology. The study was approved by ethical hospital committee to be performed from July 2016 till September 2018. The total number of admitted cases of Leiomyoma, with a clinical diagnosis and confirmed postoperatively with a histological pathology, were 385. About 244 of Leiomyoma were managed with hysterectomy (63.4%). Open myomectomy was the method of choice to treat 141 cases, which contribute to (36.4%), a different technique used, Hysteroscopic, laparoscopic or open depending on the age of the patients, location, type of leiomyoma and fertility preservation. A number of cases treated with open surgery were 70 out of 141 (49.6%) and laparoscopic myomectomy were 51 out of 141 (36.2%); only 20 cases had hysteroscopic resection of myoma (14.2%). Although hysterectomy is not an acceptable method of treatment for leiomyoma by many patients, still it is the most common surgical method for the treatment of leiomyoma.

Keywords: leiomyoma, myomectomy, hysterectomy

1. Introduction

Uterine fibroids are called uterine leiomyoma. It is one of the primary causes of morbidity in women of reproductive age [1].

It is of unknown aetiology. Several factors attribute to underlay the development and incidence of these common tumours. The fibroid is hormone-dependent, and it is known that it is a mono-cellar disease (formed from a single cell) [2].

Pathology uterine leiomyoma grossly appears as solid, white, well-circumscribed round, and not encapsulated and shows whorled appearance on the histological section. The size varies as small as microscopic to a large considerable size [3].

In 25–30% of females, fibroids are diagnosed mostly as asymptomatic [3, 4]. It is one of the primary causes of irregular vaginal bleeding, menorrhagia and metrorrhagia, and it can cause infertility, repeated abortions and a variety of pain and pressure symptoms [1].

Hysterectomy and myomectomy have been the modality used for symptomatic fibroids. In recent years, medical treatment as well as laparoscopic and hysteroscopic procedures contribute too many myoma and some other modalities.

Hysterectomy is the most frequent surgical procedure for management of leiomyomas, but the removal of leiomyoma alone is called myomectomy leaving the uterus in place; this is the second most common treatment for this condition.

The dilemma of choosing the right procedure depends on several factors: the age of the patient, size of the tumour, and fertility preservation. Fibroid frequency is diagnosed and treated; there are uncertainties and controversies among clinicians and women regarding the best way to manage them [5].

Complications of leiomyoma depend on the location of the fibroids. They can be a cause of irregular bleedings or continuous bleedings for a long time, and can also cause pain or constant pain, dysuria, constipation, and chronic bladder and bowel spasms. Rarely, they can be a cause of peritonitis. Infertility and recurrent abortion can be one of the presentations [6].

Hysterectomy is not an acceptable method of treatment of leiomyoma by many patients. The objective is to review the methods of treatment for all the cases diagnosed as leiomyoma at the Tertiary Teaching Hospital.

2. Methods

2.1 Settings and design

This is a retrospective study, data collected from medical files of all cases diagnosed as leiomyoma at King Abdulaziz University Hospital. It is a teaching hospital with a capacity of 800 beds in total and 180 beds in the Department of Obstetrics and Gynecology. The study was approved by ethical hospital committee to be performed from July 2016 till September 2018.

2.2 Data collection

The source was the medical record file, including the clinical and pathological diagnosis of leiomyoma, the surgical techniques of management, which include hysterectomy, open myomectomy, laparoscopic, and hysteroscopic myomectomy performed at King Abdulaziz University Hospital (KAUH).

2.2.1 Inclusion criteria

All patients were admitted with a diagnosis of benign leiomyoma and managed at KAUH. Exclusion criteria cases were found to be malignant or transferred to another facility, or if we found their chart was incomplete they were excluded from the analysis.

2.2.2 Statistical analysis

The Statistical Package for the Social Sciences (PC SPSS) was used to analyse data using different methods of statistical analysis.

3. Results

The total number of admitted cases of leiomyoma, with a clinical diagnosis and confirmed postoperatively with a histological pathology, were 385.

About 244 of Leiomyoma were managed with hysterectomy (63.4%). Myomectomy was the method of choice to treat 141 cases which contribute to (36.4%), a different technique used, Hysteroscopic, laparoscopic or open depending on the age of the patients, location, type of Leiomyoma, and fertility preservation.

Procedure	Number of cases	Percentage
Myomectomy	141	36.6
Hysterectomy	244	63.4
Total number	385	100

Table 1.
Total number of cases diagnosed as leiomyoma and method of treatment.

Myomectomy	Number of cases	Percentage
Open myomectomy	70	49.6
Laparoscopic myomectomy	51	36.2
Hydroscopic myomectomy	20	14.2

Table 2.
Number and percentage of the technique used for myomectomy.

A number of cases treated with open surgery were 70 out of 141 (49.6%), laparoscopic myomectomy were 51 out of 141 (36.2%), and only 20 cases had hysteroscopic resection of myoma (14.2%) (**Tables 1** and **2**).

4. Discussion

In our study, 63.4% of leiomyoma patients were treated with hysterectomy. There are many options for management of leiomyoma, which is increasing, so patients should be counselled about these options.

Not only medical and surgical managements are available, but also other modalities such as endometrial ablation and uterine artery embolization are available (**Figure 1**). Choosing an appropriate management should be based on the evidence to support specific procedures and treatments.

Here I am only listing the option of medical treatments which can be offered to women who prefer to preserve their uterus, and if conservative management indicated: medication, such as gonadotropin-releasing hormone agonists and progesterone hormone therapy, and other therapies, such as the selective oestrogen receptor modulator (raloxifene) or non-steroidal anti-inflammatory drugs [7].

A combination of MRI and ultrasonography high-intensity sound waves on the tumour, inducing coagulation necrosis can be used. Uterine artery embolisation and Myolysis, or Myolysis and endometrial ablation may reduce the need for subsequent procedures in patients with persistent bleeding.

5. Surgery

Surgery is the removal of leiomyoma only or removal of the whole uterus; and this is needed if severe symptoms exist or if leiomyoma fails to respond to other modalities. If the myoma is very small or is not causing any symptoms, usually we do not require any treatment.

Guidelines of ACOG for the management of leiomyoma exist in the literature with the risks and benefits of each option.

One of the significant factors in choosing the method of treating myoma is not only the skill of the surgeon, but also the experience of the centre in different available techniques.

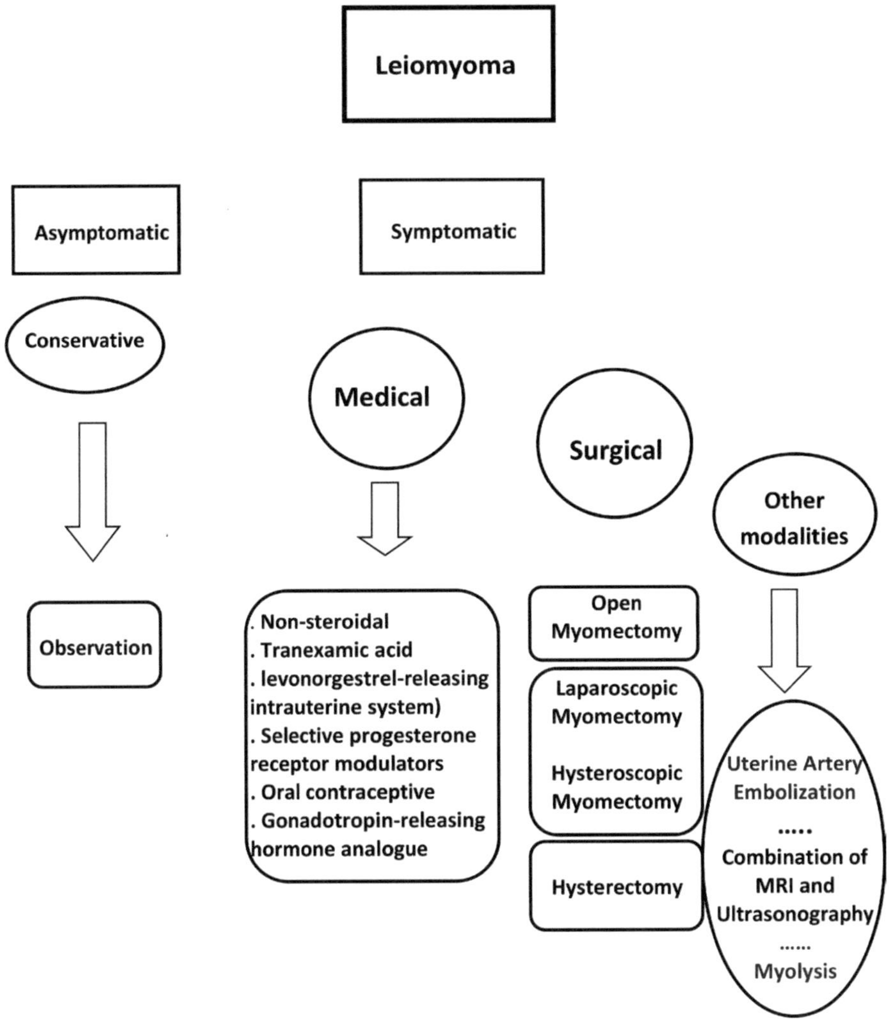

Figure 1.
Scheme of management of leiomyoma.

Hysterectomy can be done in different ways, vaginal or abdominal; depending on the technique used, the procedure can be carried out using either general or regional (a spinal-epidural) anaesthesia [6].

In many prospective studies, there was an effort taken to reduce the frequency of abdominal hysterectomy, and conclude that all patients should be counselled in detail about the alternatives to hysterectomy so that they can share the decisions [8].

Vaginal hysterectomy versus abdominal hysterectomy; in a nine RCTs, 762 women [3, 7]. It was found that the surgical approach to hysterectomy, the abdominal has more complications than other modalities; so the decision should be discussed with the patient.

6. Myomectomy

Myomectomy is considered as an alternative to hysterectomy for the treatment of leiomyoma, especially in patients who need to preserve their fertility.

Open myomectomy is useful in cases with multiple myomas, more than five and larger than 10 cm especially if deeply located.

Preoperative evaluation of the size and number of myomas is mandatory to reduce intraoperative and postoperative complications [9].

Up to 33% of women who have undergone this surgery will need a repeat procedure because of recurrence of fibroids [10].

Laparoscopic myomectomy cases may become difficult if bleeding occurs. It might need more time and longer operative time and may require for morcellation and extensive laparoscopic suturing [11].

Gynecologists need to improve their laparoscopic skills. Laparoscopic Myomectomy was associated with rapid recovery less blood and minimal postoperative pain, and fewer overall complications, but longer operating times, when compared with open myomectomy for patients with fibroids [12].

Major complications, recurrence, and pregnancy were similar between treatments. Depending on the personal experience and available equipment, the gynaecologist has a choice of several alternative procedures [13, 14].

In addition, one prospective randomised study [15] has provided good-quality evidence that surgical therapy (hysteroscopic myomectomy) yields higher pregnancy rates than alternative treatments in women with submucous myoma [16].

Acknowledgements

The work was not supported or funded by any drug company.

Conflict of interest

All authors have no conflict of interests.

Author details

Hassan S.O. Abduljabbar[1*] and Abdullah K. Agabawi[2]

1 Department of Obstetrics and Gynecology, Medical College, King Abdulaziz University, Jeddah, Kingdom of Saudi Arabia

2 Obstetrics and Gynecology Department, King Abdulaziz University Hospital, Jeddah, Saudi Arabia

*Address all correspondence to: profaj17@yahoo.com

References

[1] Li D et al. Incidence and clinical characteristics of unexpected uterine sarcoma after hysterectomy and myomectomy for uterine fibroids: A retrospective study of 10,248 cases. OncoTargets and Therapy. 2015;**8**:2943

[2] Chu J, Coomarasamy A. Myomectomy: Multiple large fibroids. In: Gynecologic and Obstetric Surgery. John Wiley & Sons; 2016. pp. 282-283

[3] Aarts JW et al. Surgical approach to hysterectomy for the benign gynecological disease. In: Cochrane Database of Systematic Reviews. 12 Aug 2015;(8):CD003677. DOI: 10.1002/14651858.CD003677.pub5

[4] Park Y-H et al. Patient-tailored self-management intervention for older adults with hypertension in a nursing home. Journal of Clinical Nursing. 2012;**22**(5-6):710-712

[5] Stewart EA. Clinical practice. Uterine fibroids. The New England Journal of Medicine. 2015;**372**(17):1646-1655. DOI: 10.1056/NEJMcp1411029

[6] Mas A et al. Updated approaches for management of uterine fibroids. International Journal of Women's Health. 2017;**9**:607-617

[7] Fenlon E, Spies JB. Nonsurgical option for fibroid treatment. In: Fibroids. Chapter 7. Wiley Online Library; 2013. pp. 76-84. https://doi.org/10.1002/9781118456996. ch 7 Cited by: 1

[8] Parker W. The utility of MRI for the surgical treatment of women with uterine fibroid tumors. American Journal of Obstetrics and Gynecology. 2012

[9] Chen B et al. Comparison of vaginal and abdominal hysterectomy: A prospective non-randomized trial. Pakistan Journal of Medical Sciences. 2014;**30**(4):875-879

[10] Neis KJ et al. Hysterectomy for benign uterine disease. Deutsches Ärzteblatt International - Online. 2016;**113**(14):242-249

[11] A U, Sanyal U. Comparison of risk of abdominal hysterectomy versus myomectomy in the management of uterine fibroids: A comparative study. International Journal of Reproduction, Contraception, Obstetrics and Gynecology. 2016;**5**(5):1345-1347

[12] Ghazali WHW et al. Five-year lapsed: Review of laparoscopic myomectomy versus open myomectomy in Putrajaya Hospital. Gynecology and Minimally Invasive Therapy. 2018;**7**(4):161

[13] Kotani Y et al. Recurrence of uterine myoma after myomectomy: Open myomectomy versus laparoscopic myomectomy. Journal of Obstetrics and Gynaecology Research. 2017;**44**(2):298-302

[14] Walid MS, Heaton RL. The role of laparoscopic myomectomy in the management of uterine fibroids. Current Opinion in Obstetrics and Gynecology. 2011;**23**(4):273-277

[15] Casini B. Bonheur et violence. Journal Le Philosophoire. 2006;26(1):77

[16] Donnez J, Dolmans M-M. Uterine fibroid management: From the present to the future. Human Reproduction Update. 2016;**22**(6):665-686

Chapter 4

New Hysteroscopic Approaches to Uterine Fibroids

Razvan Socolov, Ioana Pavaleanu, Demetra Socolov, Mona Akad and Ciprian Ilea

Abstract

The hysteroscopic myomectomy is a very important application of the gynecologic endoscopy, as it allows minimal invasive removal of the type 0, 1, and 2 fibroids with minimal damage to the uterine wall. In the last decade, new developments of this method allowed an even less invasive approach, with possibility of ambulatory procedure. We discuss the importance of these new developments, based very much on the pseudocapsule of the myoma, and analyze the literature data regarding the outcome. The cold loop resection is a technique that could be used in type 1 and type 2 myomas, with less complications and limitations than the classical electrical resectoscope. Another development, more useful for type 0 and 1 myoma, is the hysteroscopic morcellator, similar to the laparoscopic one, but providing a faster and safer procedure. We also update the complications of hysteroscopic myomectomy and their management, including long-term and obstetrical complications related to hysteroscopic myomectomy. In conclusion, new developments and studies show that hysteroscopic myomectomy has become a valid endoscopic technique ready to be used by many specialists.

Keywords: hysteroscopy, myomectomy, morcellator, cold loop resection, complications

1. Introduction

Since 1976, the fibroids were accessible to hysteroscopic approaches as a conservative treatment, especially for type 0 and type 1 of the European Society of Gynaecological Endoscopy (ESGE) classification [1]. But the instruments needed an approach requiring anesthesia and dilatation, exposing to numerous complications, especially when using monopolar electric energy. Further developments, like miniaturization of resectoscopes or the large introduction of bipolar energy, have opened new and more accessible approaches with more and more specialists using the hysteroscopic techniques and with lesser and lesser complications.

The recent years have brought a revolution in operative hysteroscopy, and myoma treatment benefitted as well as other intrauterine pathologies. We will try to point some of these developments and their applications in fibroid treatment.

2. Limits for office hysteroscopic myomectomy

The myomas are fibrotic tumors of the myometrium, with an incidence varying a lot in function of different factors (age, race, family background, etc.). Their particular structure has an outside pseudocapsule, which makes the myomectomy through enucleation a rather simple technique in laparoscopy. For the fibroids protruding into the uterine cavity (except the complete intracavitary type 0 ones), although the capsule exists, the classical approach involved a slicing technique which could impair also the surrounding myometrium, which is something not to be desired especially in young patients that want to retain a good reproductive prognostic.

The introduction of bipolar smaller resectoscopes allowed a more targeted technique. The new resectoscopes have an outer diameter of 7 mm, and this allows minimal dilatation and anesthesia. Another possibility is the bipolar probe which allows myolysis and separation from the pseudocapsule.

The use of the pseudocapsule has several advantages:

- The myoma can "move" in between the myometrial fibers, allowing its persistence during uterine contractions. During the intervention, this constitutes a cleavage plan that allows enucleation.

- Once disrupted, this pseudocapsule does not "protect" the myoma, and uterine contractions expel the tumor toward the cavity. This principle was described by as the auto-expulsion of the myoma—defined as the Office Preparation of Partially Intramural Uterine Myoma (OPPIUM) by Bettocchi et al. [2], which leaves the intramural part of the fibroid untreated in the first step. After the next menstrual cycle, the protrusion allows the hysteroscopist to resect the rest of the tumor.

This latest element is recommended in tumors exceeding 1.5 cm and with a large implantation (type 1 or type 2). Although it generally requires a two-step intervention, it offers security and facilitates the favorable final result.

Other limits to office hysteroscopic are [3]:

- Patient's sensitivity to pain, which may require some form of paracervical anesthesia and/or preoperative analgesic and antispasmodic drugs.

- The type of fibroid. Beside the cited ESGE classification, another classification is the STEP-W, which was proposed for submucous myomas by Lasmar et al. [4] and takes into account:

    - Size—largest diameter of the nodule in cm (scored as 0 if <2 cm, 1 if 2–5 cm, and 2 if >5 cm).

    - Topography in the uterine cavity (inferior part, 0; middle uterus, 1; and upper part, 2).

    - Extension of the base of the fibroid and proportion in which it covers the corresponding uterine wall (scored as 0 if <1/3, 1 if 1/3–2/3, and 2 if >2/3).

    - Penetration in the uterine wall—corresponding to the ESGE classification (0, 1, or 2 type scored as such)

    - Attachment of the fibroid to the lateral wall—if present add 1 point.

- The final score of STEP-W suggests the complexity of the case: if 0–4, easy to perform hysteroscopic myomectomy; 5–6, complex procedure, possible two-step approach; and 7–9, difficult case, and the specialist should consider alternatives to hysteroscopy.

If the myoma remains enucleated and free in the uterine cavity, there are authors that advocate leaving it for spontaneous expulsion, in the Haimovich series (after laser myomectomy) the median duration to expulsion being 68 days, with no complication [5].

An important help for better assessing the pseudocapsule could be brought by computer-aided imaging. A recent study of Török et al. [6] showed a very good accuracy, of more than 86%, using fully convolutional neural networking and high-resolution endoscopic image, which is promising for faster and safer future resections.

3. Assisting hysteroscopic myomectomy: preparation and safety

The hysteroscopic myomectomy is a method depending highly on several factors, some related to the patient (tumor size and number, consistency, position) and some to the equipment and experience of the gynecologist.

So, it is important that the preparation and safety are tackled with care.

One of the preparatory methods is the pre-treatment of fibroids. Several strategies have been proposed, and here we will discuss especially the new ones:

a. Ulipristal acetate, an orally active selective progesterone receptor modulator, could act through different mechanisms on myoma cells, inducing apoptosis, changing the expression of pro-angiogenic proteins, and reducing the production of collagen tissue. All these actions are obtained without significantly diminishing the estrogen level, unlike other therapies (i.e., GnRH agonists). According to a systematic review by Ferrero et al. [7], there are advantages and disadvantages in prescribing this treatment before hysteroscopic myomectomy. The favorable effects are the amenorrhea and diminished size of the fibroid, which would facilitate the resection. On the other hand, the endometrium appears to increase, which could create difficulties for visualization. Another mentioned change under medical pre-treatment of myomas is the "myoma migration" which means that the position and the type of fibroids could change after therapy and therefore change the approach of the surgeon, from hysteroscopy to laparoscopy and vice versa. As mentioned, this effect was also noted in the ulipristal-treated group [8] as well as in those treated by GnRH analog or embolization [9].

b. Regarding the effect of GnRH analog, the effects on the facility and duration of the hysteroscopic procedure is uncertain. As mentioned above, and in other studies [10], most of the time, for type 2 myomas, the difference was not significant in favor of the pre-treated group, but most of the series in literature are rather small. As for other types of myomas, as no important volume decrease was found, it should be emphasized that the only major advantage of the pre-treatment is reducing or stopping the associated hemorrhage.

c. For the safety increase of the procedure, the use of ultrasound vaginal scan has been shown to be of the greatest value. This allows estimation of the operating time; for example, in a study by Isono et al. [11], using the cubic value for the average diameter of the myoma was useful both in estimating the total weight of the tumor and the operating time, with differences from those with diameter of 1–2, 2–3, or >3 cm). During the procedure, the ultrasound scan has been proposed by Korkmazer et al. [12], for assessing the limits of the remaining myometrial tissue after resection of type 1 and especially type 2 myomas.

d. The 5 mm limit for safety from the serosa is the most accepted one for a safe procedure diminishing the risk of perforation [13]. Although this was considered a proven fact, new researches underline that the moment of assessing could influence this parameter. The limited use of electric energy, accompanied by squeezing the myoma from its pseudocapsule by hydro-pressure fluctuation, and other pharmacological means could, according to Casadio et al. [14], allow myomectomies of tumors with <5 mm security margin.

4. Cold loop resection: principles and limits

With this procedure, the slicing done by electrical energy is replaced by a mechanical dislocation assisted by the "natural" myometrial reaction to uterine distension that helps push the tumor toward the uterine cavity.

This technique, first described by Mazzon in 1995, had overcome the limits of classical slicing technique. It has several advantages, as described by Mazzon et al. [15]:

- Less uterine perforations, as the mechanical energy allows the myometrial tissue to contract.
- Sparing the myometrial fibers diminishes the hemorrhage associated, as it allows the natural hemostasis done by myometrial contraction and avoids damaging tortuous vessels in the deep myometrium.
- Diminishing vascular injuries also decrease the risk of distension media intravasation.
- The intramural component of the myoma loses its importance and allows smaller myoma-serosa interface than the 5 mm limit.
- The postoperative occurrence of intrauterine adhesions, a common complication of large hysteroscopic myomectomies, is also lower after cold loop technique.

The retrospective study of Mazzon [16] of 1244 cases showed a 87% of one step myomectomy in general, and 82% for type 2 myoma. Other series also allowed large myomas of >3 cm to be resected in one step by this technique, with an operating time of 10–58 min [17].

In conclusion, the cold loop method offers advantages compared to the classical electrical resectoscope one, and although it requires getting used to the use of mechanical dissection of the tumor from its pseudocapsule, with appropriate force and angle of insertion of the loop, it could have important benefit especially for large and intramural fibroids—type 1 and 2.

5. Myomectomy using hysteroscopic morcellation

The morcellation of fibroids is a technique involving mechanical cutting of small slices of tumor, accompanied by powerful suction of the fragments. The sectional mechanical effect is done, similar to laparoscopic morcellator, by rotation of an inner tube into an outer tube at high speed. The advantages of the technique, as mentioned in a large multicentric study coordinated by Scheiber et al. [18], are:

- A high efficacy, of 87% for fibroids and 99% for polyps
- The accessibility of the procedure, with similar results in ambulatory and clinical settings
- The high satisfaction of operators, up to 95%
- Low complication rate, as no repeated insertion is needed as in resectoscopic technique

A systematic review done by Vitale et al. [19] confirms the feasibility of the different morcellators in practice, especially for type 0 and 1 myomas, while type 2 myomas are more difficult, with multistep procedures, as for classical resectoscopic method. The diminished operating time, with an average of 22 min for over 280 patients in the included articles, is also an advantage.

An observation made by the authors of the cited review is that, due to the aspiration system of tissues, a larger quantity of fluid is needed. If, in classical resectoscopic myomectomy, the limit of 1000–1500 ml deficit should not be passed, in morcellating technique, even at 2500 ml deficit there was no side effect mentioned. Nevertheless, the mean deficit was much lower, around 760 ml.

Another recent prospective study of Maheux-Lacroix et al. [20] analyzed the follow-up for post-hysteroscopic morcellation patients for an average of 32 months and found a 12% rate of hysterectomies and 27% of additional surgery overall. The most significant factor for this outcome was the size of the myoma >5 cm, with odds ratio (OR) of 2.9.

There is a tendency of reducing the size of the morcellator; the new equipment with a diameter of 19 Fr (6.5 mm) allows minimal dilation and ambulatory procedures. Although this latest instrument is more suitable for polyps, Bigatti et al. [21] describes a case with type 2 fibroid resected with this shaver.

6. Postoperative follow-up and complications

6.1 Postoperative follow-up

The immediate postoperative care for patients having undergone hysteroscopic myomectomy includes surveillance of symptoms such as cramping, light bleeding, and vaginal discomfort.

The drugs of choice for postoperative pain control are usually acetaminophen or nonsteroidal anti-inflammatories. After discharge, patients are advised to use an anti-inflammatory medication such as ibuprofen, which should provide adequate pain control. Severe pain that does not respond to such medication can be a sign of a more serious complication and should be promptly evaluated.

Postoperative surveillance is further dependent upon the course of the procedure. If an imbalance of fluid was noted, then the patient should be monitored for signs and symptoms of fluid overload and hyponatremia: bradycardia, hypertension, nausea, vomiting, seizures, pulmonary edema, or cardiovascular abnormalities.

Routine activities are generally resumed within 24 h, and patients should follow standard postoperative instructions for gynecologic procedures.

Patients should be informed about further vaginal bleeding, which is anticipated for ~1 week after the surgery. The duration of bleeding may vary from a few days to 2 weeks, and the flow usually is very light.

A follow-up visit should be scheduled to take place 4–6 weeks postoperatively, when subsequent complications might be diagnosed and the pathology results reviewed and discussed with the patient, especially since cases of unexpected uterine malignancy in women undergoing hysteroscopic myomectomy were reported, with an incidence of 0.86% [22].

6.2 Complications

Operative hysteroscopy is generally considered a safe and minimally invasive procedure used for the treatment of uterine leiomyoma. Knowledge of early and late adverse events, alongside preventative measures, is crucial for the safety and quality of hysteroscopic surgery [23].

Studies regarding hysteroscopic myomectomy procedures report a complication rate of 0.8–2.6% [24, 25].

A retrospective study regarding the follow-up of 235 women with submucous fibroids at outpatient hysteroscopy who underwent a hysteroscopic transcervical resection reports a complication rate of 2.6%, and the rate is lower for procedures involving single versus multiple fibroids (1.4 vs. 6.7%) [24].

Among the gynecological procedures performed by hysteroscopy, myomectomy imposes a lower risk for complications: adhesiolysis carries the highest risk of complications (4.5%), followed by endometrial resection (0.8%), myomectomy (0.8%), and polypectomy (0.4%), as shown by a prospective study of 2515 operative hysteroscopies [25].

The most common complications of hysteroscopic myomectomy can be divided into early complications, such as uterine perforation, fluid overload, heavy bleeding, infection, and late complications and suboptimal outcomes, such as incomplete resection and intrauterine adhesions [23].

One of the most frequent complications of operative hysteroscopy is uterine perforation, with an incidence of 0.12–3% [24–26]. The incidence increases in the presence of risk factors for traumatic entry: menopausal status, cervical stenosis, retroversion, and nulliparity. Signs and symptoms of uterine perforation include a sudden increase in fluid deficit and loss of adequate intracavitary distention, which generally results in loss cavitary distention, leading to termination of the procedure. Nevertheless, it can result in bleeding and potentially significant injury to surrounding organs, depending mainly on the type of instrument used.

If the perforation was caused by a blunt instrument during dilation of the cervix, it can be managed conservatively if major bleeding is not suspected. In these cases of suspected uterine perforation without hemodynamic instability and suspicion of damage to major vessels, postoperative monitoring of red blood cell count is essential, and a single dose of prophylactic antibiotic may be considered [23].

Damage by electrosurgical electrodes may lead to more serious injuries [27]. In this case, if a thermal or mechanical injury to surrounding viscera is suspected, a diagnostic laparoscopy is necessary.

In the long term, uterine perforation is a potential cause of uterine rupture in pregnancy which should not be neglected [28].

The incidence of fluid overload during operative hysteroscopy ranges between 1.6 and 2.5%, making excess fluid absorption one of the most common complications associated with hysteroscopic procedures [29].

The term "operative hysteroscopy intravascular absorption syndrome" (OHIA) was introduced, regarding the excessive fluid overload caused by intravasation of distension media [23, 30], which further leads to hyponatremia and volume overload [3] and, in severe cases, metabolic acidosis, pulmonary and cerebral edema, and severe OHIA being associated with a mortality of 25% [30].

Continuous fluid monitoring, as well as thoughtful consideration of the distention media used, is an essential measure in preventing fluid overload. Isotonic media and bipolar equipment are preferred in order to reduce the risk of hyponatremia and its consequences [23]. Recent guidelines by the British Society of Gynaecological Endoscopy (BSGE) and the European Society of Gynaecological Endoscopy on fluid management in operative hysteroscopy recommend an upper threshold of 2500 ml for isotonic media and for of 1000 ml hypotonic fluids, in healthy women [31]. For patients with comorbidities or at an advanced age, lower thresholds are recommended: fluid deficit levels of 750 ml for hypotonic solutions and 1500 ml for isotonic solutions [31].

Heavy bleeding is uncommon after operative hysteroscopy but might occur due to mechanical trauma to the endometrium and/or myometrial vessels. Management options include intracervical injection of a prostaglandin F2α analog, resulting in uterine contraction with subsequent decrease in uterine bleeding or an intracavitary placement of a Foley catheter with a 30-ml balloon providing counterpressure. The balloon can be deflated, and the Foley removed after the bleeding has subsided for 4 hours. In rare cases, the bleeding may persist and require uterine arterial embolization or hysterectomy [23].

The incidence of infection following operative hysteroscopy varies between 0.01 [5] and 1.42% [32]. Prevention of infection may be possible by reducing the duration of the intervention. Currently, there is no established role for prophylactic antibiotic use.

Attention should be given to the possibility of postoperative uterine adhesion formation, especially in patients with a desire for future fertility. This complication is more likely to occur when lesions on opposing uterine walls have been resected so that the surfaces are juxtaposed after the procedure is completed. In these instances, estrogen therapy could be utilized immediately postoperatively, causing a rapid development of the endometrium. Another method attempted in the past was the placement of an intrauterine Foley catheter to prevent the contact between the opposing surfaces. Performing a hysteroscopy 6 weeks after surgery can be helpful both for diagnosis and for treatment by blunt dissection of adhesions with the tip of the hysteroscope [33].

Although rare, cases with abnormal placentation following hysteroscopic resection of myomas have also been reported. In 2013, Mathiesen et al. have reported the first case of placenta increta (associated with placenta previa) in a pregnancy after hysteroscopic myomectomy, concluding that patients with a history of hysteroscopic myomectomy are at an increased risk for abnormal placentation [34]. Tanaka et al. have reported in 2016 a case of placenta accreta without placenta previa during a pregnancy subsequent to hysteroscopic myomectomy, which was obtained with cryopreserved embryo transfer, which has been reported as an independent risk factor for placenta accreta. The authors suggest that any patient with previous hysteroscopic myomectomy should be considered to be at high risk for placenta accreta, even if she does not develop placenta previa [35].

Regarding the efficacity of hysteroscopic treatment of myomas, studies show a high success rate of hysteroscopic resection of uterine leiomyoma, of >94% [24], depending on prognostic factors such as the size, location, and number of myomas. The incidence of incomplete resection rates ranges from 5 to 20.5% [23, 36]. Reinterventions are usually performed, but may not always be necessary [23]. Comorbid conditions such as adenomyosis or dysfunctional uterine bleeding can result in persistent menorrhagia that may indicate a subsequent hysterectomy for definitive treatment.

7. Conclusion

The hysteroscopic myomectomy has benefitted from the technical developments in equipment, and things appear to continue. Both new instrumentations and a more physiological approach to the myoma enucleation could be increasing the safety and the efficacy of this type of procedures.

Conflict of interest

The authors declare no conflict of interest.

Author details

Razvan Socolov*, Ioana Pavaleanu, Demetra Socolov, Mona Akad and Ciprian Ilea
Department of Obstetrics and Gynecology, University of Medicine and Pharmacy Gr T Popa, Iasi, Romania

*Address all correspondence to: socolov.razvan@gmail.com

References

[1] Wamsteker K, Emanuel MH, de Kruif JH. Transcervical hysteroscopic resection of submucous fibroids for abnormal uterine bleeding: Results regarding the degree of intramural extension. Obstetrics and Gynecology. 1993;**82**:736-740

[2] Bettocchi S, Di Spiezio Sardo A, Ceci O, Nappi L, Guida M, Greco E, et al. A new hysteroscopic technique for the preparation of partially intramural myomas in office setting (OPPIuM technique): A pilot study. Journal of Minimally Invasive Gynecology. 2009; **16**:748-754. DOI: 10.1016/j.jmig.2009.07.016

[3] Lasmar RB, Lasmar BP. Chapter 35. Limiting factors of office hysteroscopic myomectomy. In: Tinelli A, Pacheco LA, Haimovich S, editors. Hysteroscopy. Cham: Springer International Publishing; 2018. pp. 357-363. DOI: 10.1007/978-3-319-57559-9

[4] Lasmar RB, Barrozo PR, Dias R, Oliveira MA. Submucous myomas: A new presurgical classification to evaluate the viability of hysteroscopic surgical treatment-preliminary report. Journal of Minimally Invasive Gynecology. 2005;**12**:308-311. DOI: 10.1016/j.jmig.2005.05.014

[5] Haimovich S, López-Yarto M, Urresta Ávila J, Saavedra Tascón A, Hernández JL, Carreras Collado R. Office hysteroscopic laser enucleation of submucous myomas without mass extraction: A case series study. BioMed Research International. 2015;**2015**: 905204. DOI: 10.1155/2015/905204

[6] Török P, Harangi B. Digital image analysis with fully connected convolutional neural network to facilitate hysteroscopic fibroid resection. Gynecologic and Obstetric Investigation. 2018;**83**:615-619. DOI: 10.1159/000490563

[7] Ferrero S, Vellone VG, Barra F, Scala C. Ulipristal acetate before hysteroscopic and laparoscopic surgery for uterine myomas: Help or hindrance? Gynecologic and Obstetric Investigation. 2018;**14**:1-13. DOI: 10.1159/000495347

[8] Willame A, Marci R, Petignat P, Dubuisson J. Myoma migration: An unexpected "effect" with ulipristal acetate treatment. European Review for Medical and Pharmacological Sciences. 2016;**20**:1439-1444

[9] Wen L, Tseng JY, Wang PH. Vaginal expulsion of a submucosal myoma during treatment with long-acting gonadotropin-releasing hormone agonist. Taiwanese Journal of Obstetrics & Gynecology. 2006;**45**:173-175

[10] Favilli A, Mazzon I, Grasso M, Horvath S, Bini V, Di Renzo GC, et al. Intraoperative effect of preoperative gonadotropin-releasing hormone analogue administration in women undergoing cold loop hysteroscopic myomectomy: A randomized controlled trial. Journal of Minimally Invasive Gynecology. 2018;**25**:706-714. DOI: 10.1016/j.jmig.2017.11.011

[11] Isono W, Wada-Hiraike O, Sugiyama R, Maruyama M, Fujii T, Osuga Y. Prediction of the operative time for hysteroscopic myomectomy for leiomyomas penetrating the intramural cavity using leiomyoma weight and clinical characteristics of patients. Reproductive Medicine and Biology. 2018;**17**(4):487-492. DOI: 10.1002/rmb2.12228

[12] Korkmazer E, Tekin B, Solak N. Ultrasound guidance during hysteroscopic myomectomy in G1 and G2 submucous myomas: For a safer one step surgery. European Journal of Obstetrics, Gynecology, and

Reproductive Biology. 2016;**203**: 108-111. DOI: 10.1016/j.ejogrb.2016. 03.043

[13] Litta P, Leggieri C, Conte L, Dalla Toffola A, Multinu F, Angioni S. Monopolar versus bipolar device: Safety, feasibility, limits and perioperative complications in performing hysteroscopic myomectomy. Clinical and Experimental Obstetrics & Gynecology. 2014;**41**(3):335-338

[14] Casadio P, Guasina F, Talamo MR, Magnarelli G, Mazzon I, Seracchioli R. Chapter 38. Is the distance between myoma and serosa a limiting factor? In: Tinelli A, Pacheco LA, Haimovich S, editors. Hysteroscopy. Cham: Springer International Publishing; 2018. pp. 387-401. DOI: 10.1007/978-3-319-57559-9

[15] Mazzon I, Favilli A, Villani V, Gerli S. Chapter 36. Hysteroscopic myomectomy respecting the pseudocapsule: The cold loop hysteroscopic myomectomy. In: Tinelli A, Pacheco LA, Haimovich S, editors. Hysteroscopy. Cham: Springer International Publishing; 2018. pp. 387-401. DOI: 10.1007/978-3-319-57559-9

[16] Mazzon I, Favilli A, Grasso M, Horvath S, Bini V, Di Renzo GC, et al. Predicting success of single step hysteroscopic myomectomy; a single center large cohort study of single myomas. International Journal of Surgery. 2015;**22**:10-14. DOI: 10.1016/j.ijsu.2015.07.714

[17] Di Spiezio SA, Calagna G, Di Carlo C, Guida M, Perino A, Nappi C. Cold loops applied to bipolar resectoscope: A safe "one-step" myomectomy for treatment of submucosal myomas with intramural development. The Journal of Obstetrics and Gynaecology Research. 2015;**41**(12):1935-1941. DOI: 10.1111/jog.12831

[18] Scheiber MD, Chen SH. A prospective multicenter registry of patients undergoing hysteroscopic morcellation of uterine polyps and myomas. Journal of Gynecologic Surgery. 2016;**32**(6):318-323

[19] Vitale SG, Sapia F, Rapisarda AMC, Valenti G, Santangelo F, Rossetti D, et al. Hysteroscopic morcellation of submucous myomas: A systematic review. BioMed Research International. 2017;**2017**:6848250. DOI: 10.1155/2017/6848250.

[20] Maheux-Lacroix S, Mennen J, Arnold A, Budden A, Nesbitt-Hawes E, Won H, et al. The need for further surgical intervention following primary hysteroscopic morcellation of submucosal leiomyomas in women with abnormal uterine bleeding. The Australian & New Zealand Journal of Obstetrics & Gynaecology. 2018;**58**: 570-575. DOI: 10.1111/ajo.12781

[21] Bigatti G, Ansari SH, Di W. The 19 Fr. Intrauterine Bigatti shaver (IBS®): A clinical and technical update. Facts, Views & Visions in ObGyn. 2018;**10**(3): 161-164

[22] Yuk J-S, Shin J-Y, Moon H-S, Lee JH. The incidence of unexpected uterine malignancy in women undergoing hysteroscopic myomectomy or polypectomy: A national population-based study. European Journal of Obstetrics, Gynecology, and Reproductive Biology. 2018;**224**:12-16. DOI: 10.1016/j.ejogrb.2018.03.003

[23] Aas-Eng MK, Langebrekke A, Hudelist G. Complications in operative hysteroscopy: Is prevention possible? Acta Obstetricia et Gynecologica Scandinavica. 2017;**96**:1399-1403. DOI: 10.1111/aogs.13209

[24] Polena V, Mergui JL, Perrot N, Poncelet C, Barranger E, Uzan S. Long-term results of hysteroscopic myomectomy in 235 patients. European

Journal of Obstetrics, Gynecology, and Reproductive Biology. 2007;**130**(2): 232-237. DOI: 10.1016/j.ejogrb.2006.01.014

[25] Jansen FW, Vredevoogd CB, van Ulzen K, Hermans J, Trimbos JB, Trimbos-Kemper TC. Complications of hysteroscopy: A prospective, multicenter study. Obstetrics and Gynecology. 2000;**96**(2):266-270. DOI: 10.1016/S0029-7844(00)00865-6

[26] Aydeniz B, Gruber IV, Schauf B, Kurek R, Meyer A, Wallwiener D. A multicenter survey of complications associated with 21676 operative hysteroscopies. European Journal of Obstetrics, Gynecology, and Reproductive Biology. 2002;**104**: 160-164. DOI: 10.1016/S0301-2115(02)00106-9

[27] Propst A. Complications of hysteroscopic surgery: Predicting patients at risk. Obstetrics and Gynecology. 2000;**96**:517-520. DOI: 10.1016/S0029-7844(00)00958-3

[28] Sentilhes L, Sergent F, Roman H, Verspyck E, Marpeau L. Late complications of operative hysteroscopy: Predicting patients at risk of uterine rupture during subsequent pregnancy. European Journal of Obstetrics, Gynecology, and Reproductive Biology. 2005;**120**: 134-138. DOI: 10.1016/j.ejogrb.2004.10.010

[29] Hahn RG. Fluid absorption in endoscopic surgery. British Journal of Anaesthesia. 2006;**96**:8-20. DOI: 10.1093/bja/aei279

[30] Sethi N, Chaturvedi R, Kumar K. Operative hysteroscopy intravascular absorption syndrome: A bolt from the blue. Indian Journal of Anaesthesia. 2012;**56**:179-182

[31] Umranikar S, Clark TJ, Saridogan E, Miligkos D, Arambage K, Torbe E, et al. BSGE/ESGE guideline on management of fluid distension media in operative hysteroscopy. Gynecological Surgery. 2016;**13**:289-303. DOI: 10.1007/s10397-016-0983-z

[32] Agostini A, Cravello L, Shojai R, Ronda I, Roger V, Blanc B. Postoperative infection and surgical hysteroscopy. Fertility and Sterility. 2002;**77**:766-768. DOI: 10.1016/S0015-0282(01)03252-6

[33] Dongen HV, Emanuel MH, Smeets MJ, Trimbos B, Jansen FW. Follow-up after incomplete hysteroscopic removal of uterine fibroids. Acta Obstetricia et Gynecologica Scandinavica. 2006;**85**: 1463-1467. DOI: 10.1080/00016340600984647

[34] Mathiesen E, Hohenwalter M, Basir Z, Peterson E. Placenta increta after hysteroscopic myomectomy. Obstetrics and Gynecology. 2013;**122**: 478-481. DOI: 10.1097/AOG.0b013e31828aef0a

[35] Tanaka M, Matsuzaki S, Matsuzaki S, Kakigano A, Kumasawa K, Ueda Y, et al. Placenta accreta following hysteroscopic myomectomy. Clinical Case Reports. 2016;**4**:541-544. DOI: 10.1002/ccr3.562

[36] Emanuel MH, Wamsteker K, Hart AA, Metz G, Lammes FB. Long-term results of hysteroscopic myomectomy for abnormal uterine bleeding. Obstetrics and Gynecology. 1999;**93**:743-748. DOI: 10.1016/S0029-7844(98)00558-4

Chapter 5

Uterine Fibroid Embolization

Said Izreig, Arash Fereydooni and Naiem Nassiri

Abstract

Uterine fibroids or leiomyomas are benign, hormone-dependent smooth muscle cell tumors that can be associated with menorrhagia, anemia, pelvic pain, urinary and/or intestinal symptoms, and dyspareunia. Traditionally, the mainstay of treatment has been surgical, consisting of hysterectomy or myomectomy. However, uterine artery embolization has become an increasingly utilized, minimally invasive treatment modality that can be offered as either sole therapy or as a staged, pre-operative measure to hysterectomy. A thorough knowledge of pelvic vascular anatomy and facility with specific embolotherapeutic techniques are required for safe and effective fibroid embolization.

Keywords: uterine artery embolization, uterine fibroid, embolic agent, menorrhagia, internal iliac artery

1. Introduction

Uterine fibroids (UF), or leiomyomas, are benign tumors arising from uterine smooth muscle. UF are common with reported lifetime prevalence rates approaching 70% in Caucasian women and over 80% in African American women [1]. Symptomatic fibroids—estimated to comprise less than 50% of all UF—are most commonly associated with menorrhagia and subsequent anemia in women of reproductive age [2]. As UF grow in volume, symptoms related to bulk effects, including constipation, bladder dysfunction, tenesmus, and chronic back and pelvic pain become problematic and may warrant intervention.

Controversy exists regarding the effect of UF on fertility. Several systematic reviews have reported evidence of increased rates of spontaneous abortion and decreased fertility [3, 4]. Because these reviews included numerous studies drawn from populations of women seeking reproductive assistance, the results presented may not be generalizable to all reproductive-aged women. A systematic review of studies drawn from general obstetric populations found no relation between risk of spontaneous abortion and presence of UF [5].

The traditional approach to UF management has been surgical. Hysterectomy remains the predominant intervention, with myomectomy an option for women desiring to maximize fertility. Uterine artery embolization (UAE) is a minimally invasive and uterine preserving procedure that has become an attractive therapeutic alternative over the last 20 years. Its efficacy and acceptable safety profile have helped establish the technique as a viable approach with minimal complications for women interested in retaining their uterus and avoiding invasive surgery [6]. The procedure involves percutaneous transarterial catheterization and embolization of the vessels perfusing the UF in an attempt to induce ischemic necrosis of the culprit lesion(s).

2. Risk factors and pathophysiology

The exact etiology of UF remains unclear. Several factors are thought to contribute to the overall risk of developing UF, including black race, nulliparity, advanced age prior to menopause, obesity, and hypertension [7, 8]. Menarche before age 10 and oral contraceptive use are also associated with increased risk [7, 9]. Bleeding and bulk symptoms associated with UF tend to ameliorate with menopause, suggesting that the persistence of UF depends on hormonal status [2]. There also exists a hereditary component, with first degree relatives of women affected by UF having a 2.5 fold higher risk of developing UF [10]. Recurrent chromosomal alterations and genetic mutations are found in a fraction of all UF [11, 12]. Protective factors include multiparity, a well-balanced diet, and progestin-only injectable contraception [7, 9, 13].

UF are classified based on their extent and location within the uterus. Broadly, submucosal fibroids are found immediately below the endometrium; subserosal fibroids beneath the serosal uterine surface; intramural fibroids within the myometrium; and pedunculated fibroids are suspended from the uterus by a stalk and may project into the peritoneal or uterine cavities. The International Federation of Obstetrics and Gynecology classification system describes UF localization on an eight-point scale with lower values denoting closer fibroid proximity to the endometrium and uterine cavity [14].

Submucosal fibroids carry an additional risk of endocavitary expulsion post-UAE [15]. Those with larger endometrial interface to maximum dimension ratio are even more likely to be completely or partially expelled into the uterine cavity. In general, larger masses are associated with higher complications rates, although the majority of endocavitary masses pass with few symptoms [15]. For women whose UF fit the above profile and wish to undergo UAE, explaining the risk and symptomatology of fibroid expulsion is essential to minimize post-procedural distress and ensure prompt engagement with their physician should expulsion manifest.

3. Imaging

Identification of UF is often incidental to pelvic examination or pelvic imaging. In patients with suggestive symptoms, trans-abdominal or trans-vaginal ultrasound is initially performed [16]. Color flow Doppler interrogation of the mass can help delineate the degree of vascularity of the UF. B-mode imaging can help delineate the location, depth, extent, and configuration of the UF. Further details of the uterine mass, including presence of potential malignancy, vascularization patterns and anastomoses, and the risk for passage of the infarcted mass, can be captured using contrast-enhanced MRI. Importantly, pre-procedural MRI provides a baseline measure of perfusion that can be tracked to measure the degree of infarction post-UAE [17–19]. It is important to note that imaging ought to be performed in coordination with a thorough gynecologic evaluation and examination including endometrial biopsy to rule out other etiologies. A multidisciplinary approach to patient care in close collaboration with colleagues in gynecology can lead to excellent outcomes [20].

4. Indications and patient selection

Asymptomatic UF discovered incidentally can generally be managed non-operatively under the supervision of a gynecologist. Women experiencing symptomatic UF, however, are candidates for intervention and should be counseled regarding the options available to them. Numerous guidelines have described the best practices for UAE based on reported clinical evidence [21]. A consistent picture regarding the ideal candidate for UAE is presented across guidelines: a patient with symptomatic fibroids (bleeding, pain, mass effects) who wishes to avoid invasive surgery. Frequently reported absolute contraindications include viable pregnancy and active infection [21]. Commonly cited relative contraindications include immunocompromised status, hostile anatomy for endovascular intervention, renal impairment, contrast allergy, or previous uterine surgery.

Variability exists among guidelines regarding relative contraindications. Several guidelines recommend considering some UF as unsuitable for UAE based on the relative position of the mass in the uterus; with pedunculated, submucosal and subserosal fibroids variably suggested as being unsuitable for UAE [21–24]. Other guidelines make no such recommendations regarding UF positioning, leaving the anatomical suitability of a patient for UAE at the discretion of the treating physician [21, 25]. Patient desire to retain fertility is similarly divisive. Some guidelines cite a small reported advantage in fertility outcomes of women treated with myomectomy compared to UAE as rationale for recommending against UAE in women desiring future fertility [26, 27]. Other studies have demonstrated similar rates of fertility and complications associated with pregnancy in women treated with UAE when compared with the general population [28, 29]. Definitive evidence regarding the effects of UAE on fertility remains outstanding. It is our practice to recommend against UAE in patients wishing to maintain fertility [20].

Larger UF measuring greater than 10 cm or large uteruses greater than 24 weeks were once considered contraindications to UAE based on case reports detailing poor outcomes in women bearing these features [30]. Continued research and experience, however, has demonstrated the safety and efficacy of UAE for treatment of large UF and large uteruses [31, 32]. We currently do not recommend against UAE based on UF or uterine size alone [20].

The determination of the best treatment approach for a given patient with UF should begin with a consultation that covers a complete history and physical, a review of OB/GYN examination and assessment, the type and degree of symptoms, and a review of any available imaging. Ascertaining the patient's desire for future fertility and uterus preservation are important considerations in guiding intervention selection. In cases where UAE is indicated, explaining the risks associated with the procedure, including bleeding, infection, access site complications, possible negative effects on fertility and the potential need for surgical reintervention and hysterectomy, offers the patient a full account on which to base their decision.

Though rare, other indications for UAE include abnormal placental development, such as placenta previa, accreta, increta, and percreta. These conditions are commonly treated by emergency hysterectomy and carry a high risk of intrapartum hemorrhage, respiratory distress syndromes, kidney failure, and death. Hybrid prophylactic bilateral UAE and caesarian section has been described to increase the safety of fetus delivery and to minimize the risk of intrapartum hemorrhage from placental detachment [33]. In a hybrid operating room, bilateral uterine arteries are first cannulated and the infant is delivered. While the umbilical cord is clamped and the vaginal cavity is packed with the placenta in situ, both uterine arteries are embolized. In a series of 12 patients who underwent UAE-assisted cesarean section, 10 patients retained their uterus and 2 underwent hysterectomy [33]. There was no mortality, minimal blood loss and no post-operative infection. In these cases, the risk of low dose radiation to the fetus is considered negligible compared with baseline risks for all developmental abnormalities [34]. UAE may fall under the purview of multiple specialties, and a collaborative effort among gynecologists, interventional radiologists, and vascular surgeons is necessary to expand the availability of UAE and/or other surgical measures to more women [20].

5. Vascular anatomy of the female pelvis

It is vital to delineate the normal vascular anatomy and its variations for prevention of non-target embolization. In its most common configuration (77%), the internal iliac artery (IIA) bifurcates into two main stems, one anterior and one posterior. Other modes of IIA division include three-stem in 14%, four- or more-stem in 3%, and one main stem in 4% of cases. The anterior division branches include the obturator, umbilical/superior vesical, uterine, vaginal, inferior vesical, middle hemorrhoidal, inferior gluteal, and internal pudendal arteries. The posterior trunk gives rise to the iliolumbar, the lateral sacral, and the superior gluteal arteries. The superior gluteal artery is invariably the terminal branch. While the iliac bifurcation and the origin of the IIA is best visualized under contralateral anterior oblique projection, we have found ipsilateral anterior oblique projections to best demonstrate the origin and course of the uterine artery once the IIA has been adequately accessed and catheterized [35].

The diameter of the uterine artery varies from 2 to 5 mm and is usually largest during pregnancy and immediately after childbirth. It has a U-shaped course. It initially courses caudally against the pelvic wall, then horizontally across the ureter, and at last cranially along the uterus. Its three major terminal branches are the artery of uterine fundus, medial tubal branch, and medial ovarian artery. It is important to be aware of the medial ovarian branch coursing along the utero-ovarian ligament, as it anastomoses with a branch originating from the ovarian artery. The medial ovarian branch provides the total ovarian supply in 4% of the cases. Uterine artery branches are extensively anastomosed with the contralateral uterine artery, as well as with the ipsilateral ovarian and the inferior epigastric arteries. While the uterine artery provides most of the arterial supply of the uterus, the ovarian artery and the artery of the round ligament also contribute [36].

UF are not fed by a specific branch, but by a peri-myomatous plexus. In the presence of fibroids, the branches of the uterine artery are distorted and larger in caliber [16]. The superficial surface of UF are usually enveloped in a dense perifibroid arterial plexus whereas the core of the mass remains relatively hypovascular [16, 37]. The ovarian arteries contribute to UF arterial supply in 5–10% of the cases, especially in patients who have disturbed arterial networks secondary to prior pelvic surgery, tubal or ovarian pathologies or a large fundal fibroid. Round ligament arteries and lumbar arteries are rare sources of UF perfusion. Left–right uterine artery anastomoses are identified in roughly 10% of patients and ovarian-uterine artery anastomoses in 10–30% [16]. On the contrary, pedunculated fibroids are generally perfused by a solitary artery coursing through the fibrotic stalk. A proposed risk of necrosis and deterioration of the stalk with liberation of the mass into the peritoneal cavity has been used as a justification for classifying pedunculated fibroids as a relative contraindication to UAE [38]. Nevertheless, contrast-enhanced magnetic resonance imaging (MRI) of pedunculated fibroids treated with UAE found intact vascularization of the peduncle stalk with successful infarction of the mass and no complications related to UF location [38]. Other work has suggested that pedunculated fibroids are less likely to be completely infarcted following UAE although no clinical outcome data were reported [39]. The suitability of UAE in the treatment of pedunculated fibroids remains an outstanding issue. We currently do not recommend against UAE in patients with pedunculated UF configurations.

6. Choice of embolic agent

An array of embolic particles has been developed and employed in clinical practice. One of the earliest embolic materials used was non-spherical polyvinyl alcohol particles (nsPVA; Merit Medical, South Jordan UT). nsPVA are non-uniform in size and shape and are, therefore, dependent on thrombus formation to produce complete occlusion of the uterine artery lumen [40]. nsPVA also tends to occlude microcatheters and complicate delivery. MRI assessment of UF treated with UAE using nsPVA frequently showed recanalization of infarcted UF in a majority of women 6 months post-intervention, highlighting the need for newer embolic agents suited for UAE [41]. Thus, spherical polyvinyl alcohol (sPVA) particles were developed to address the size and shape variation of nsPVA; however, in practice, sPVA particles (Contour SE microspheres; Boston Scientific) produced inferior improvements in symptoms and smaller reductions in UF size post-UAE [42].

Gelatin sponge—a biodegradable agent derived from purified gelatin—has been used as an embolic agent in cases of hemorrhage, and has been employed successfully as an embolic agent in UAE [43]. Preparing the gelatin sponge agent from the stock material requires hand manipulation, which produces inconsistencies in size and shape thereby limiting quantifiable comparisons with other more consistently prepared embolic agents.

Particle size influences the degree of distal embolization and potential for non-target embolization [31]. The observed caliber of perifibroid arterial vessels is between 500 and 800 μm, which justifies the typical use of calibrated particles in the 500–700 or 700–900 μm range [44]. Employing smaller sized particles is associated with an increased risk of uterine necrosis and should therefore be avoided [45].

Tris-acryl gelatin microspheres (TAGM; Embospheres; Merritt Medical, South Jordan, Utah) are calibrated microspheres that come in sizes ranging from 40 to 1200 μm. When used for UAE, TAGM sized 500–700 μm are typically employed and have demonstrated distal penetration into the UF vasculature with minimal proximal aggregation that is observed with nsPVA [40].

A new entrant in the embolic material space is F-coated Hydrogel Microspheres Embozene; CeloNova BioScience, Newnan, Georgia. These microspheres are comprised of a hydrogel core of polymethylmethacrylate encased in a malleable polyphosphazene shell. These particles are biostable and are available in a range of sizes from 40 to 1300 μm [40]. Early experience with these agents has demonstrated safety and efficacy in the treatment of UF [46].

With the exception of greater symptomatic improvement with TAGM use as compared to sPVA, outcomes and complications of the other embolic agents generally suggests no clear evidence of superiority of TAGM [40, 42]. There is a need for better powered studies to differentiate among the different embolic agents.

7. Technical procedure

UAE is generally performed in a hybrid operating suite or catheterization suite under general or moderate sedation anesthesia. The latter requires ability and willingness of the patient to cooperate with positional and ventilatory instructions intraoperatively to maximize imaging quality as well as the accuracy of microcatheterization and embolic agent delivery. In the absence of contraindications, chemical and mechanical deep vein thrombosis prophylaxis via prophylactic dose of enoxaparin, graded stockings, and sequential compressive devices is administered before induction of anesthesia.

The single femoral artery approach is adequate to access both the ipsilateral and contralateral uterine arteries. The micropuncture technique is used for femoral arterial access. In young healthy women, clinically significant vasospasm is a serious consideration and must be monitored regularly. We suggest immediate availability of vasodilatory agents for intrarterial administration if necessary. In order to avoid arterial vasospasm, some interventionalists recommend ceasing GnRH analog treatment several weeks before treatment [20, 35].

Over a guidewire, a 5 F multisidehole catheter of choice is advanced into the midabdominal aorta. Flush aortography is performed looking for pelvic hypervascular neoplastic changes and dilation and tortuosity of the feeding UAs. Contralateral obliquity of the image intensifier facilitates visualization of the ipsilateral iliac bifurcation. Under roadmap guidance, selective catheterization of the IIA is performed using an angled guidewire and a 5 F C2 catheter (Merit Medical, South Jordan UT). Selective angiogram of the IIA in ipsilateral obliquity commonly facilitates visualization of the UA ostium. This image is then roadmapped. A coaxial microcatheter-based platform (Direxion; Boston Scientific, Marlborough, MA) is then developed over an 0.014 steerable guidewire, the tip of which can be curved manually before intrarterial insertion to help facilitate engagement of the target vessel ostium and to help overcome extreme arterial tortuosity.

Superselective microcatheterization of the UA is then performed with advancement of the catheter to the proximal-most branches of the uterine artery feeding the fibroid. Use of power injector for angiography is essential as manual contrast infusion through the small caliber, high resistance microcatheter platform can be difficult and lead to suboptimal imaging. Once the satisfactory positioning of microcatheter tip is confirmed on angiography, the system is copiously flushed with heparinized saline in preparation for the delivery of embolic agent [20].

The embolic agent is delivered in bursts through the microcatheter under fluoroscopic guidance with intermittent heparin saline flush. Extreme care is taken to avoid reflux of the embolic agent particularly toward the end of each session when greater resistance to flow is encountered. The system is then gently flushed with heparinized saline to irrigate out the residual embolic content within the microcatheter. This must be performed under fluoroscopic visualization to prevent nontarget embolization. Adequate devascularization of the UF from the accessed side is then confirmed on completion angiography of the ipsilateral IIA through the 5 F C2 catheter after removing the microcatheter coaxial platform.

Up-and-over technique is used to similarly catheterize the contralateral UA and deliver embolic agent as described previously. Completion aortoiliac angiogram is performed to ensure adequate UF devascularization and to rule out nontarget embolization.

Alternative techniques have been reported. Bilateral femoral puncture with sequential UA catheterization and simultaneous embolization is associated with reduced fluoroscopy time, reduced procedure time, and no added complication risk when compared to unilateral femoral puncture [47]. Transradial access (TRA) has been employed successfully in percutaneous coronary interventions for years, and studies exploring the suitability of TRA for UAE have been promising [48, 49]. In those patients with sufficient collateral perfusion of the hand and suitable radial artery anatomy, TRA may have 100% technical success rate with no immediate complications [49]. Patients usually enjoy fewer restrictions in positioning and movement following the procedure and report satisfaction with the freedom offered by TRA.

8. Outcomes and complications

Accumulated evidence over decades has supported the use of UAE in the treatment of uterine masses in a safe and efficacious manner. Expected outcomes following UAE include a 50–60% reduction in UF size, an 88–92% reduction in bulk symptoms associated with UF, 90% reduction in bleeding associated symptoms, and a patient satisfaction rate of 80–90% [25, 26]. Reduction in UF size can be visualized within weeks of UAE and continues for 3–12 months following the procedure. Histopathological analysis of successfully infarcted UF is characterized by coagulative or hyaline necrosis [50]. The degree of UF infarction as captured by contrast enhanced MRI 24–72 hours post-UAE has been reported to predict the magnitude and durability of symptomatic improvement as well as risk for reintervention [51]. Women exhibiting 100% infarction on post-operative imaging enjoyed a 0% reintervention rate after 24 months, whereas women with almost complete (90–99%) or partial (<90%) infarction experienced reintervention rates of 20 and 50%, respectively.

Interventional success is generally defined as reducing blood flow through the UA to near stasis and causing complete infarction of the UF [6]. Gradual revascularization of the myometrium occurs in the weeks following UAE while the UF ideally remains infarcted and regresses. Failure rates range from 20 to 28%, most likely due to incomplete embolization of the UF vasculature, recanalization of the UF vasculature, or the persistence and engorgement of collaterals feeding the UF post-UAE [6, 52]. Identification of collateral blood supply to the UF, either before UAE using an aortogram or MRI, or peri-procedurally using cone-beam CT angiography, will inform the embolization procedure and ensure all vessels supplying the UF are targeted [6, 53]. In cases where the ovarian artery is found to supply the UF, either independently or via a utero-ovarian anastomosis, embolization of the ovarian artery is required to ensure complete infarction of the UF. Despite the risk of ovarian compromise following ovarian artery embolization in this scenario, reports studying the effects of ovarian artery embolization in conjunction with UAE have found no evidence of menopause precipitation, nor worsening of menopausal symptoms [52]. This is in contrast to prior work that reported roughly 40% of women over the age of 45 experienced ovarian failure following UAE without ovarian artery embolization [54]. Among women under the age of 45, no cases of ovarian failure were observed. These observations suggest that, should UAE negatively affect the ovarian capacity, the extent of ovarian function compromise is related to the patient's age at the time of the procedure.

Post-embolization syndrome, involving pelvic pain, low-grade fever, nausea, loss of appetite, and malaise, is almost inevitable following UAE. The treatment is supportive, consisting of antipyretic, fluids, analgesia, and anti-inflammatory medication. Over 90% of women undergoing UAE report pain following the procedure, making pain management an important consideration in caring for these patients [55]. Admitting patients for a 24-hour observation period allows for pain management under the direct care of their physician. [20] Several approaches have been reported that aim to reduce post-procedural pain and opioid use in these patients. Peri-procedural superior hypogastric nerve block using a 0.75% ropivacaine solution is effective in minimizing post-procedural pain and significantly reduces total opioid usage [55]. A single pre-procedural dose of intravenous dexamethasone can also improve patient pain scores and reduce markers of inflammation. However, the total opioid use in these patients has been found not to be significantly different from those not receiving pre-procedural dexamethasone [56].

The most commonly reported long-term complication associated with UAE is permanent amenorrhea. Women over 45 years of age are reported more likely to experience permanent amenorrhea following UAE (20–40%) than women under 45 (0–3%) [25]. Transient amenorrhea following UAE is often observed and may be a consequence of non-target ovarian artery embolization although this is not considered a major complication. Other observed complications include persistent vaginal discharge, transcervical expulsion of infarcted tissue, prolonged and intractable pain, and infection [25]. Very rare cases of deaths have been reported following

UAE as a result of pulmonary embolization, sepsis, and embolization of occult leiomyosarcoma [31].

Reintervention is indicated, should UF related symptoms return secondary to resumed growth of the primary UF or growth of a new UF. Reported reintervention rates range from 14 to 35% [26, 57]. Reinterventions may include repeat UAE, hysterectomy, or myomectomy. Patients undergoing UAE should be counseled regarding the risks of reintervention. Fostering long-term relationships with patients undergoing UAE allows for tracking of outcomes and early intervention should symptoms re-emerge [25].

While several guidelines cite preservation of fertility as a relative contraindication to UAE, uncertainty remains regarding fertility outcomes following the procedure [21]. Published case series following pregnancies in women attempting to conceive following UAE found an overall pregnancy rate of ~30% [58]. As compared to the general obstetric population, women treated with UAE have similar or increased rates of obstetric complications, with specifically increased rates of miscarriage and cesarean section deliveries [58, 59]. Notably in the majority of these studies, women with UF treated by UAE were older than the general obstetric population and carried additional risk factors, which may explain some of the observed increases in complication rates. For women with complex UF pathology who desire to retain their uterus and avoid invasive surgery, UAE may be presented as an option that preserves some chance of conception in the future.

9. Comparison with hysterectomy and myomectomy

The traditional approach to the treatment of symptomatic fibroids has been surgical, with hysterectomy being the most common [60]. Complete removal of the uterus is a definitive treatment for UF that precludes recurrence and may be a suitable recommendation for women who have completed child bearing. Though rates of hysterectomy are decreasing, the lifetime prevalence among U.S women as of 2012 was 45%, with nearly one-third of all hysterectomies performed as treatment of UF [60]. While laparoscopic hysterectomy has become more commonplace, open hysterectomies remain most frequently employed.

Myomectomy is a uterine sparing surgical intervention best suited to the removal of one to three fibroids in an anatomically accessible location [31]. Like hysterectomy, myomectomy may be done laparoscopic or open, with the laparoscopic approach associated with fewer complications and quicker recovery [61]. For women with submucosal fibroids projecting into the intrauterine cavity, hysteroscopic myomectomy is a suitable option that is associated with quick recovery and return to daily living [2].

Laparoscopic management of UF, either by hysterectomy or myomectomy that employs power morcellation for specimen removal, has been associated with a risk of dissemination of occult sarcoma [31]. Histopathological analysis of hysterectomy specimens shows a 0.4% rate of unsuspected malignancy in uteruses treated for UF [62]. Under these circumstances, patients should be informed of the risk of occult malignancy dissemination.

Growing clinical experience and promise of UAE in the treatment of UF motivated the design and execution of several randomized clinical trials (RCTs) comparing medium- and long-term outcomes and patient satisfaction with UAE compared with surgical interventions. The embolization versus hysterectomy (EMMY) trial recruited women with symptomatic UF and assigned them 1:1 to either UAE or hysterectomy [63]. Patient satisfaction rates and quality of life scores were similar between UAE and hysterectomy out to 10 years [64]. The study reported a 69% success rate with UAE while 31% of UAE treated patients experienced refractory or relapsing symptoms requiring definitive treatment by hysterectomy. Of note was the observation that women with BMI >25 and a history of smoking at baseline were more likely to require reintervention following UAE. The reported 69% clinical success rate is notably lower than other reported rates ranging 80–90% [31]. The authors attributed the lower UAE success rate to the fact that eligible candidates recruited to the study suffered severe bleeding symptoms, and the trial required a much longer 10-year follow-up window that is only used in tracking outcomes [64].

The REST trial grouped women treated with myomectomy with women treated with hysterectomy in order to expand the UAE comparison to surgical intervention [65]. Women treated with either UAE or surgery enjoyed similar satisfaction rates and quality of life improvements at 5 years. Differences in reintervention rates were noted, however, as 32% of women treated with UAE required further intervention within 5 years as compared to 4% of women in the surgery group. A study directly comparing UAE to myomectomy found symptom improvement in 88.3% of UAE women compared to 75.4% in myomectomy at 2 years post-intervention [66]. Bearing the risks of reintervention in mind, the above trials affirm UAE as a safe procedure that enjoys rates of satisfaction and symptom improvement similar to those observed in hysterectomy and myomectomy. A Cochrane review of published RCTs comparing UAE to surgical interventions reaffirms this view and shows that UAE is associated with shorter hospital stays, less disability, and similar satisfaction rates when compared to surgical intervention [26].

10. New generation of devices

Magnetic resonance-guided high intensity focused ultrasound (MR-g HIFU) is a non-invasive intervention that works to thermally ablate UF via the delivery focused ultrasound waves [67]. Rounds of sonification and heating lasting 30 seconds are interleaved with 90-second cooling-off periods; the target tissue temperatures reach 60–85°C, thereby provoking coagulative necrosis of the targeted mass [68]. FDA guidelines regarding MR-g HIFU limit the total and percent volumes of uterine mass subject to thermal ablation to confine the sonification to the fibroid. Prospective studies tracking symptom severity scores and quality of life indices in women, whose UF were treated with MR-g HIFU, found significant improvement of both measures after at least 2 years of follow-up [67, 68]. In a direct comparison with UAE, however, women who underwent MR-g HIFU reported smaller improvements to quality of life scores after treatment [69]. MR-g HIFU also fared worse in terms of reintervention rates, with women undergoing UAE experiencing a 6.7% reintervention rate compared to a 30% reintervention rate in the MR-g HIFU group at mid-term follow up [69]. Potential explanations for the different outcomes are that MR-g HIFU treats only a single mass whereas UAE targets all masses in the uterus, and that MR-g HIFU ablates only a fraction of the total mass volume whereas UAE completely infarcts UF.

11. Conclusion

As the rates of hysterectomy fall and patient desire for less invasive management of uterine fibroid rises, uterine artery embolization has become increasingly prominent. Two decades of experience have validated the procedure as safe and effective with continued advancement in procedural techniques, equipment and imaging, embolic agents, pain management, and operator experience lending to improved outcomes. There remain outstanding questions regarding UAE. Well-controlled investigations of fertility outcomes in women undergoing UAE or surgery for UF are needed. As new embolic agents become available, comparison trials to gauge efficacy and safety among the different agents are necessary. Continued delineation of patient anatomy that suggest susceptibility to ovarian insufficiency post-UAE is also important to ensure patients are well-counseled regarding their risks. The potential for further advancement leaves UAE well-positioned to continue its expansion in clinical practice.

Abbreviations

EMMY	embolization versus hysterectomy
F	French
MR-g HIFU	magnetic resonance-guided high intensity focused ultrasound
MRI	magnetic resonance imaging
nsPVA	non-spherical polyvinyl alcohol
RCT	randomized clinical trials
SPRM	selective progesterone receptor modulators
sPVA	spherical polyvinyl alcohol
TAGM	tris-acryl gelatin microspheres
TRA	transradial access
UAE	uterine artery embolization
UF	uterine fibroid
UPA	ulipristal acetate

Author details

Said Izreig[1], Arash Fereydooni[1] and Naiem Nassiri[2]*

1 School of Medicine, Yale University, New Haven, CT, United States

2 Department of Surgery, School of Medicine, Division of Vascular and Endovascular Surgery, Yale University, New Haven, CT, United States

*Address all correspondence to: naiem.nassiri@yale.edu

References

[1] Baird DD et al. High cumulative incidence of uterine leiomyoma in black and white women: Ultrasound evidence. American Journal of Obstetrics and Gynecology. 2003;**188**(1):100-107

[2] Stewart EA. Clinical practice. Uterine fibroids. The New England Journal of Medicine. 2015;**372**(17):1646-1655

[3] Pritts EA, Parker WH, Olive DL. Fibroids and infertility: An updated systematic review of the evidence. Fertility and Sterility. 2009;**91**(4):1215-1223

[4] Sunkara SK et al. The effect of intramural fibroids without uterine cavity involvement on the outcome of IVF treatment: A systematic review and meta-analysis. Human Reproduction. 2010;**25**(2):418-429

[5] Sundermann AC et al. Leiomyomas in pregnancy and spontaneous abortion: A systematic review and meta-analysis. Obstetrics and Gynecology. 2017;**130**(5):1065-1072

[6] Kohi MP, Spies JB. Updates on uterine artery embolization. Seminars in Interventional Radiology. 2018;**35**(1):48-55

[7] Marshall LM et al. A prospective study of reproductive factors and oral contraceptive use in relation to the risk of uterine leiomyomata. Fertility and Sterility. 1998;**70**(3):432-439

[8] Medikare V et al. The genetic bases of uterine fibroids: A review. Journal of Reproduction and Infertility. 2011;**12**(3):181-191

[9] Wise LA et al. Reproductive factors, hormonal contraception, and risk of uterine leiomyomata in African-American women: A prospective study. American Journal of Epidemiology. 2004;**159**(2):113-123

[10] Vikhlyaeva EM, Khodzhaeva ZS, Fantschenko ND. Familial predisposition to uterine leiomyomas. International Journal of Gynaecology and Obstetrics. 1995;**51**(2):127-131

[11] Makinen N et al. MED12, the mediator complex subunit 12 gene, is mutated at high frequency in uterine leiomyomas. Science. 2011;**334**(6053):252-255

[12] Ligon AH, Morton CC. Genetics of uterine leiomyomata. Genes Chromosomes and Cancer. 2000;**28**(3):235-245

[13] Wise LA et al. Intake of fruit, vegetables, and carotenoids in relation to risk of uterine leiomyomata. The American Journal of Clinical Nutrition. 2011;**94**(6):1620-1631

[14] Munro MG et al. The FIGO classification of causes of abnormal uterine bleeding in the reproductive years. Fertility and Sterility. 2011;**95**(7):2204, 2208 e1-2208, 2208 e3

[15] Verma SK et al. Submucosal fibroids becoming endocavitary following uterine artery embolization: Risk assessment by MRI. American Journal of Roentgenology. 2008;**190**(5):1220-1226

[16] Pelage JP et al. Uterine fibroid vascularization and clinical relevance to uterine fibroid embolization. Radiographics. 2005;**25** (Suppl 1):S99-S117

[17] Keung JJ, Spies JB, Caridi TM. Uterine artery embolization: A review of current concepts. Best Practice and Research. Clinical Obstetrics and Gynaecology. 2018;**46**:66-73

[18] Fleischer AC et al. Three-dimensional color Doppler sonography before and after fibroid embolization.

Journal of Ultrasound in Medicine. 2000;**19**(10):701-705

[19] Pelage JP et al. Uterine fibroid tumors: Long-term MR imaging outcome after embolization. Radiology. 2004;**230**(3):803-809

[20] Nassiri N et al. An academic tertiary referral center's experience with a vascular surgery-based uterine artery embolization program. Annals of Vascular Surgery. 2018;**52**:90-95

[21] Chen HT, Athreya S. Systematic review of uterine artery embolisation practice guidelines: Are all the guidelines on the same page? Clinical Radiology. 2018;**73**(5):507 e9-507 e15

[22] Vilos GA et al. The management of uterine leiomyomas. Journal of Obstetrics and Gynaecology Canada. 2015;**37**(2):157-178

[23] Carranza-Mamane B et al. The management of uterine fibroids in women with otherwise unexplained infertility. Journal of Obstetrics and Gynaecology Canada. 2015;**37**(3):277-285

[24] Marret H et al. Therapeutic management of uterine fibroid tumors: Updated French guidelines. European Journal of Obstetrics, Gynecology, and Reproductive Biology. 2012;**165**(2):156-164

[25] Dariushnia SR et al. Quality improvement guidelines for uterine artery embolization for symptomatic leiomyomata. Journal of Vascular and Interventional Radiology. 2014;**25**(11):1737-1747

[26] Gupta JK et al. Uterine artery embolization for symptomatic uterine fibroids. Cochrane Database of Systematic Reviews. 2014;**12**:CD005073

[27] Goldberg J et al. Pregnancy outcomes after treatment for fibromyomata: Uterine artery embolization versus laparoscopic myomectomy. American Journal of Obstetrics and Gynecology. 2004;**191**(1):18-21

[28] Pisco JM et al. Pregnancy after uterine fibroid embolization. Fertility and Sterility. 2011;**95**(3):1121 e5-1121 e8

[29] Mohan PP, Hamblin MH, Vogelzang RL. Uterine artery embolization and its effect on fertility. Journal of Vascular and Interventional Radiology. 2013;**24**(7):925-930

[30] Pelage JP et al. Fibroid-related menorrhagia: Treatment with superselective embolization of the uterine arteries and midterm follow-up. Radiology. 2000;**215**(2):428-431

[31] Silberzweig JE et al. Management of uterine fibroids: A focus on uterine-sparing interventional techniques. Radiology. 2016;**280**(3):675-692

[32] Berczi V et al. Safety and effectiveness of UFE in fibroids larger than 10 cm. Cardiovascular and Interventional Radiology. 2015;**38**(5):1152-1156

[33] Li Q et al. Prophylactic uterine artery embolization assisted cesarean section for the prevention of intrapartum hemorrhage in high-risk patients. Cardiovascular and Interventional Radiology. 2014;**37**(6):1458-1463

[34] Patel SJ et al. Imaging the pregnant patient for nonobstetric conditions: Algorithms and radiation dose considerations. Radiographics. 2007;**27**(6):1705-1722

[35] Varghese K, Adhyapak S. Uterine artery embolization for bleeding due to fibroids. In: Therapeutic Embolization. Cham: Springer International Publishing; 2017. pp. 83-92

[36] Boyer L et al. Uterine fibroid embolization (UFE). In: Chabrot P, Boyer L, editors. Embolization. London: Springer London; 2014. pp. 323-340

[37] Goodwin SC, Spies JB. Uterine fibroid embolization. The New England Journal of Medicine. 2009;**361**(7):690-697

[38] Smeets AJ et al. Safety and effectiveness of uterine artery embolization in patients with pedunculated fibroids. Journal of Vascular and Interventional Radiology. 2009;**20**(9):1172-1175

[39] Lacayo EA et al. Leiomyoma infarction after uterine artery embolization: Influence of embolic agent and leiomyoma size and location on outcome. Journal of Vascular and Interventional Radiology. 2017;**28**(7):1003-1010

[40] Das R et al. Comparison of embolic agents used in uterine artery embolisation: A systematic review and meta-analysis. Cardiovascular and Interventional Radiology. 2014;**37**(5):1179-1190

[41] Das R et al. MRI assessment of uterine artery patency and fibroid infarction rates 6 months after uterine artery embolization with nonspherical polyvinyl alcohol. Cardiovascular and Interventional Radiology. 2013;**36**(5):1280-1287

[42] Rasuli P et al. Spherical versus conventional polyvinyl alcohol particles for uterine artery embolization. Journal of Vascular and Interventional Radiology. 2008;**19**(1):42-46

[43] Katsumori T, Kasahara T, Akazawa K. Long-term outcomes of uterine artery embolization using gelatin sponge particles alone for symptomatic fibroids. American Journal of Roentgenology. 2006;**186**(3):848-854

[44] Siskin GP et al. Leiomyoma infarction after uterine artery embolization: A prospective randomized study comparing tris-acryl gelatin microspheres versus polyvinyl alcohol microspheres. Journal of Vascular and Interventional Radiology. 2008;**19**(1):58-65

[45] Pelage JP et al. Uterine artery embolization in sheep: Comparison of acute effects with polyvinyl alcohol particles and calibrated microspheres. Radiology. 2002;**224**(2):436-445

[46] Smeets AJ et al. Embolization of uterine leiomyomas with polyzene F-coated hydrogel microspheres: Initial experience. Journal of Vascular and Interventional Radiology. 2010;**21**(12):1830-1834

[47] Costantino M et al. Bilateral versus unilateral femoral access for uterine artery embolization: Results of a randomized comparative trial. Journal of Vascular and Interventional Radiology. 2010;**21**(6):829-835. quiz 835

[48] Fischman AM, Swinburne NC, Patel RS. A technical guide describing the use of transradial access technique for endovascular interventions. Techniques in Vascular and Interventional Radiology. 2015;**18**(2):58-65

[49] Resnick NJ et al. Uterine artery embolization using a transradial approach: Initial experience and technique. Journal of Vascular and Interventional Radiology. 2014;**25**(3):443-447

[50] Weichert W et al. Uterine arterial embolization with tris-acryl gelatin microspheres: A histopathologic evaluation. The American Journal of Surgical Pathology. 2005;**29**(7):955-961

[51] Kroencke TJ et al. Uterine artery embolization for leiomyomas: Percentage of infarction predicts

clinical outcome. Radiology. 2010;**255**(3):834-841

[52] Hu NN et al. Menopause and menopausal symptoms after ovarian artery embolization: A comparison with uterine artery embolization controls. Journal of Vascular and Interventional Radiology. 2011;**22**(5):710-715 e1

[53] Alabdulghani F, O'Brien A, Brophy D. Application of cone-beam computed tomography angiography in a uterine fibroid embolization procedure: A case report. Case Reports in Radiology. 2018;**13**(1):130-134

[54] Chrisman HB et al. The impact of uterine fibroid embolization on resumption of menses and ovarian function. Journal of Vascular and Interventional Radiology. 2000;**11**(6):699-703

[55] Binkert CA et al. Superior hypogastric nerve block to reduce pain after uterine artery embolization: Advanced technique and comparison to epidural anesthesia. Cardiovascular and Interventional Radiology. 2015;**38**(5):1157-1161

[56] Kim SY et al. The effects of single-dose dexamethasone on inflammatory response and pain after uterine artery embolisation for symptomatic fibroids or adenomyosis: A randomised controlled study. BJOG-An International Journal of Obstetrics and Gynaecology. 2016;**123**(4):580-587

[57] Sandberg EM et al. Reintervention risk and quality of life outcomes after uterine-sparing interventions for fibroids: A systematic review and meta-analysis. Fertility and Sterility. 2018;**109**(4):698-707 e1

[58] Carpenter TT, Walker WJ. Pregnancy following uterine artery embolisation for symptomatic fibroids: A series of 26 completed pregnancies. BJOG-An International Journal of Obstetrics and Gynaecology. 2005;**112**(3):321-325

[59] Walker WJ, McDowell SJ. Pregnancy after uterine artery embolization for leiomyomata: A series of 56 completed pregnancies. American Journal of Obstetrics and Gynecology. 2006;**195**(5):1266-1271

[60] Stewart EA, Shuster LT, Rocca WA. Reassessing hysterectomy. Minnesota Medicine. 2012;**95**(3):36-39

[61] Jin C et al. Laparoscopic versus open myomectomy—A meta-analysis of randomized controlled trials. European Journal of Obstetrics, Gynecology, and Reproductive Biology. 2009;**145**(1):14-21

[62] Takamizawa S et al. Risk of complications and uterine malignancies in women undergoing hysterectomy for presumed benign leiomyomas. Gynecologic and Obstetric Investigation. 1999;**48**(3):193-196

[63] Volkers NA et al. Uterine artery embolization versus hysterectomy in the treatment of symptomatic uterine fibroids: 2 years' outcome from the randomized EMMY trial. American Journal of Obstetrics and Gynecology. 2007;**196**(6):519 e1-519 11

[64] de Bruijn AM et al. Uterine artery embolization vs hysterectomy in the treatment of symptomatic uterine fibroids: 10-year outcomes from the randomized EMMY trial. American Journal of Obstetrics and Gynecology. 2016;**215**(6):745 e1-745 e12

[65] Moss JG et al. Randomised comparison of uterine artery embolisation (UAE) with surgical treatment in patients with symptomatic uterine fibroids (REST trial): 5-year results. BJOG-An International Journal of Obstetrics and Gynaecology. 2011;**118**(8):936-944

[66] Siskin GP et al. A prospective multicenter comparative study between myomectomy and uterine artery embolization with polyvinyl alcohol microspheres: Long-term clinical outcomes in patients with symptomatic uterine fibroids. Journal of Vascular and Interventional Radiology. 2006;**17**(8):1287-1295

[67] Kim HS et al. MR-guided high-intensity focused ultrasound treatment for symptomatic uterine leiomyomata: Long-term outcomes. Academic Radiology. 2011;**18**(8):970-976

[68] Funaki K, Fukunishi H, Sawada K. Clinical outcomes of magnetic resonance-guided focused ultrasound surgery for uterine myomas: 24-month follow-up. Ultrasound in Obstetrics and Gynecology. 2009;**34**(5):584-589

[69] Froeling V et al. Midterm results after uterine artery embolization versus MR-guided high-intensity focused ultrasound treatment for symptomatic uterine fibroids. Cardiovascular and Interventional Radiology. 2013;**36**(6):1508-1513